Integrated Mathematics of Radiographic Exposure

Integrated Mathematics of Radiographic Exposure

Sandra Jones Ireland, B.A., R.T. (R)

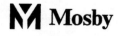 Mosby

An Affiliate of Elsevier Science

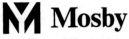

An Affiliate of Elsevier Science

Managing Editor: Jeanne Rowland
Project Manager: Peggy Fagen
Production Editor: Graphic World Publishing Services
Designer: Rita Naughton

First edition
Copyright © 1994 by Mosby, Inc.
A Mosby imprint of Mosby, Inc.

Printed in the United States of America

Mosby, Inc.
11830 Westline Industrial Drive
St. Louis, Missouri 63146

ISBN 0-8151-4834-8

/ 9 8 7 6 5 4 3 2

This book is dedicated to my husband, Bill, who patiently helped me learn how to liberate the "X" in an equation, who read many drafts of this manuscript, and who, like the students I've worked with, helped me develop a more pleasant way to teach these problems.

S.L.J.I.

Reviewers

Ken Roszel, MS, RT(R)
Clinical Instructor
School of Radiography
Geisinger Medical Center
Danville, Pennsylvania

Carri Clark-Sorensen, BS, RT(R)
Supervisor, Radiology
St. Mary's Hospital and Medical
    Center
Grand Junction, Colorado

Ron Bohland, RT(R)(M)
Clinical Coordinator
St. Charles Hospital
Oregon, Ohio

Michael Fugate, MEd, RT(R)
Faculty Member
Radiography Program
Sante Fe Community College
Gainesville, Florida

Preface

Radiographers have many challenges and responsibilities in their daily tasks. Among them is working with the complex calculations used to efficiently and safely operate x-ray generating equipment. This book is designed and written to help you as a student or practicing radiographer learn how to evaluate and solve radiographic technique problems and understand why the solutions will work.

As you hone your skills in doing the calculations and evaluating how technique changes affect the imaging process, you will find it useful to discuss the pros and cons of technique selections with your colleagues and with radiologists. You will sometimes be confronted with mathematical problems that seem almost too complex to be understood, but as you work through this book, you will find there are no mysteries in solving these problems.

Radiographers are encouraged to work with technical changes on a "one-at-a-time" basis, but often actual practice demands that multiple changes in technical factors be incorporated into calculations. These situations require the radiographer to know how each factor may affect the over-all diagnostic quality of the recorded image. These are challenges all radiographers face, and to help you, this book uses an integrated approach to solving technique problems that is student-centered and problem-based.

When I originally accepted a challenge to teach mathematics of radiographic exposure, I was placed in the ultimate problem-based learning situation. I had to come up with clear and efficient ways to explain radiographic concepts, numbers, equations and formulas in an integrated, understandable, interesting and applicable way. I discovered why, as I was told, ". . . no one else wants to teach this course."

As I developed the lecture notes for the class on mathematics of radiographic exposure, I discovered the information on technique manipulations in most books to be so cursory that several books were needed to adequately explain singular, but integrated, concepts.

Additionally, I learned another interesting, but unpublished, bit of information about the mathematics of radiographic exposure. In his unpublished ASRT Fellow Thesis, Edward C. Bressler, R.T.(R), FASRT, determined that for each technique setting, there are minimally 1,152-plus technique options. By taking his research a bit further, Bressler found that if one takes into consideration the selections of kilovoltage (kVp), milliamps-seconds (mAs), and beam collimation, the technique option combinations may number 82,000 or more (Bressler 1981).

These statistics present a staggering challenge to the student and radiographer, but with proper and understandable education and clinical experience, the radiographer is better prepared to make independent technical decisions and reasonably predict the results.

In teaching, my goals are to (1) involve the students in their learning by giving them more responsibility for that process, (2) help students understand how problems and concepts are interrelated, and (3) help them see that problems and concepts are easy to understand. These goals are reflected in the structure and content of this workbook.

With a stronger base of knowledge, the student will gain greater confidence, be willing to question, seek answers, and continue to study and learn beyond the prescribed formal educational time frame.

Some instructors tell me that students who score high on the various entrance exams, or students who have an intuitive sense of numbers and concepts, have no problem with mathematics of radiographic exposure.

While this may be true, I wonder why so many radiographers tell me they don't really understand math of exposure. I also wonder why some radiographers have difficulty selecting manual techniques or understanding how to put a term like mAs into its component parts.

This book addresses those areas of radiographic science that often require the most immediate attention and accuracy in calculations and decision-making by the radiographer. Since basic concepts are presented in this workbook and supported by additional reading, research and professional inquiry, the skills and concepts learned will work quite well in other areas such as physics, sensitometry, linear tomography and magnification, to name a few associated areas.

The structure of the book will foster a positive mentor-teaching relationship between the student and the instructor so you are partners in the learning experience.

Along my educational path, I have encountered some special people whose generosity of spirit in teaching and life has brought me a greater understanding of the importance of sharing knowledge.

I wish to thank Dr. G. F. "Bee" Hanlon, ACVR, my first mentor, who gave me encouragement and who shared her wisdom; Robert M. Lockery, R.T., FASRT, who shared his insights in teaching and taught me how to turn negative experiences into positive ones; Julia Peters who believed in me and this idea from the beginning; William P. Ireland, DVM, Ph.D., for his work in editing and evaluating this manuscript, and for sharing his expertise and enthusiasm for mathematics as a useful tool in understanding the integrated concepts of radiology; and Jeanne Rowland, my managing editor, whose enthusiasm and sense of humor gave this project a joyful vitality.

And lastly, but equally important, I thank all of the students from whom I learned the value and power of generously sharing knowledge. I am indebted to all of these people; they are exceptional individuals.

NOTE: This book on mathematics of exposure can be taught in conjunction with or without film critique sessions.

The problems in this book are presented as an aid in learning how to do and understand the subject material and come from my notes. The techniques *ARE NOT* intended to be used as techniques for radiological examinations.

Sandra Jones Ireland

Table of Contents

Integrated Mathematics of Radiographic Exposure

Introduction

Objectives

■ ■ ■ ■ ■ ■ ■ ■ ■ ■

After studying this unit, the student should be able to:

1. Define the general components of an integrated system of radiographic mathematics.

2. Discuss the importance of working with one technical factor at a time.

3. Identify and discuss a radiographer's responsibilities.

4. Discuss why the patient presents many technical challenges.

5. Discuss baseline and manual techniques and the usefulness and limitations of automatic exposure devices.

6. Identify at least two components of a student-centered approach to learning.

This unit is designed as an orientation to the structure of this book. The task of learning as much as you can about your profession may not always be easy, but it is one of the most important things you can do. On occasion, the technical information may seem difficult and hard to put into context. When this happens, check with your instructors and discuss elements that are confusing or of concern.

The mathematics of radiographic exposure is an integrated system, which means that if one factor is changed, other factors will be affected. Because of this relationship, students and practicing radiographers, and others who may work directly with the practical application of x-rays as a diagnostic tool in medicine or industry, must understand and be able to reasonably predict the effects on the resulting film when radiographic technique changes are made. Thus the following practical advice is to be taken seriously:

> ■   ■
>
> Change only one factor at a time.
>
> ■   ■

This advice is especially useful as you sharpen your mathematical skills in this specialized area, first, in the classroom, and last, while working with radiographic equipment and with patients. Of course, this advice is not always heeded, and on occasion, you will be faced with making multiple exposure factor technique decisions. If you have studied and practiced technique calculations and manipulations, you will be prepared to deal with the challenges facing you.

RADIOGRAPHER'S RESPONSIBILITIES

Specifically, an integrated system in the mathematics of radiographic exposure means that as the radiographer, you are responsible for the following:

1. Safety and comfort of the patient in your care.

2. Proper positioning of the patient, the radiographic imaging device, and associated radiographic accessories.

3. The selection of exposure factors needed to produce a diagnostic radiographic film. In selecting the techniques, the radiographer makes independent decisions based on measurements of the anatomical part or other objects to be radiographed, selects the kVp, mA, and seconds (mAs).

4. Deciding on the speed and size of the film and cassette, and grid that will be used for the procedure.

5. Selection of the Source-Image Distances (SID) to be used, and should be prepared to work with distances different from the one indicated on the technique chart. The radiographer must know and understand how distance affects the intensity of the x-ray beam, how the change in intensity affects the radiographic film, and make compensatory changes.

6. Selection of intensifying screens of different speeds, different types of stationary and reciprocating grids, types of radiographic units, and so forth. And even if the department limits these choices, the radiographer must know how to make the proper technical changes.

7. Working with and using manual technique selections despite the availability of automatic exposure devices (AED).

8. Knowledge of technical compensations for other items such as: changes in grid ratio, use of compensating filters, specialized cones or collimation, type of x-ray generator, e.g., single phase or three-phase; capacitor, battery-operated or pulsating. In addition, the radiographer must have

a thorough working knowledge of the equipment and how to use the equipment safely, efficiently, and advantageously.

9. And most important, the radiographer is responsible for the comfort and care of the patient, who is the ultimate challenge.

> THE PATIENT is the ultimate challenge in technique selection.

Professional experience has shown that the patient is perhaps the greatest variable over which we have little mathematical control.

While we can measure the thickness of the part to be radiographed as an aid in the selection of a technique, one must consider the patient's body shape, age, and general physical condition. Even so, we still must make independent technique decisions based on our observations concerning these and many other aspects of the patient.

One needs to be aware that standardized technique charts are generally designed around the optimum average patient who is ambulatory and in relatively good health. At best, a technique chart is a guide, and when used effectively, it reduces the radiation exposure to the patient, saves time, and helps reduce departmental operating expenses.

The evaluation of the patient's habitus and physical condition are variables that will take some time to learn. While you are learning to make these evaluations, you should study and refer to the many textbooks that contain information on how pathology, age, and so forth affect the attenuation of the primary beam as it passes through the patient and is recorded on the film.

TECHNIQUE CHART STANDARDIZATION

As you progress through the classes that prepare you for working with radiographic imaging equipment and the accessories, you will learn that radiographers standardize as many of the mathematical factors as possible.

In the course of learning to work with radiographic techniques, you will learn how to establish a standardized basis for those times when you are required to develop and/or tailor a technique chart for a procedure or equipment.

There was a time when many radiographers prided themselves on a so-called ability to "pull techniques out of the air." For newcomers to the profession, this ability seemed like some sort of magic that defied explanation. But you will discover in your course of study that there is no magic involved in the selection of techniques, although it seems that way.

In the past, technique charts were not always readily available, even though technique charts were often provided by the x-ray machine manufacturer.

Sometimes technique charts were displayed, usually taped to the front of the control panel, on the movable lead shielding or another convenient place near the control panel. But unfortunately, most technique charts were often kept in a desk drawer. Why did this happen?

This happened because technique charts were rarely tailored to meet the needs of the specific departments, radiographic examinations, or the interpretation needs of the radiologists.

As a result, most radiographers and students kept a personal pocket technique book that contained useful notes on techniques and positions used.

Fortunately, in most modern radiology departments, technique charts are required and must be prominently displayed and used, although I suspect that most radiographers still keep a personal notebook on useful technique tips.

EXPOSURE TECHNIQUE BASE LINES

Before you can effectively work with radiographic exposure techniques or establish a technique chart, you must know the factors assigned to accessories such as films, grids, intensifying screens, and the minimum and maximum ratings of your equipment.

With this information you are ready to standardize your radiographic and processing equipment and develop technique charts. This information will also allow you more time to focus on the variables inherent in all patients.

The objectives in setting up a technique chart are:

1. The reduction in the number of repeat exposures that will result in reduced radiation exposure to patients.

2. Standardized exposure techniques result in better quality control to help you make adjustments for nonstandardized variables.

3. Provide greater accuracy in the selection of technique changes.

There are various types of technique charts. Some of them have a fixed kVp—variable mAs or variable kVp—fixed mAs. Other charts are based on use of automatic exposure devices. But regardless of the type of technique chart used, it is imperative that the radiographer know how to accurately make adjustments in any technical factor.

There is a baseline technique formula that has been identified in many textbooks and one which many radiographers have used to begin the establishment of a technique chart.

> Starting kilovoltage = (cm thickness of the part × 2) + base kilovoltage.

The base kilovoltage can be an arbitrary number -OR- it can be the lowest kVp setting on the machine. This starting kVp number should be carefully selected. You might want to consider as criteria for the starting kilovoltage such things as the penetration of the part needed to obtain the scale of contrast and density that will adequately expose the film without compromising the safety of the patient or the limitations of major or accessory equipment.

But as with any kind of technique guide, the baseline formula must be refined specifically for your departmental needs and always with the patient in mind. Use of a phantom can be used to help you refine the radiographic techniques.

Some useful references are: Burns: 1992; Bushong: 1993; Carlton-Adler: 1992; Cullinan-Cullinan: 1994; Hiss: 1993.

AUTOMATIC EXPOSURE DEVICES (AEDs)

Modern radiographic imaging equipment generally comes with Automatic Exposure Devices (AEDs), but even so, the radiographer must have a strong understanding of the technique factors used in manual technique selection to work effectively with the AEDs.

Automatic Exposure Devices (AEDs), when used effectively, aid in reducing radiation exposure, expedite the procedure, and reduce the number of repeat films if properly used.

As a word of caution: It is easy to rely on the use of automated exposure devices, and though these devices are sophisticated and useful, the radiographer must also have a solid understanding of the mathematics of exposure, anatomy, some pathology, and contrast media studies when using the AEDs.

There will be times when an automatic exposure device is not available, especially for bedside or portable radiography, if the patient is confined to a wheelchair or a stretcher, or if the AED is not working properly. Or you may have a difficult radiographic exposure problem that is not easily solved by using an AED. In these instances expert knowledge of the manipulation of radiographic exposure factors is essential.

While a goal in mathematics of exposure may be to master the process of manipulating techniques, it is also important to understand how each factor is a part of the radiographic technique selection process.

Regardless of the easy or difficult exposure situations and problems you may face in the course of your career, it is your responsibility to be able to deal with these challenges in a professional and efficient manner.

This book is designed to help you develop your skills in the manipulation of the radiographic factors used each time you make an exposure. It is designed to help you become proficient in making the necessary calculations with greater ease and to help you understand the concepts behind the technique selection processes.

Allow yourself time to practice and experiment with the numbers, formulas, and calculations used in making technical factor adjustments. Be willing to make mistakes, on paper, of course. Practice the calculation procedures, set up new problems, and study the problems to help you become comfortable with the calculations and concepts.

STUDENT-CENTERED APPROACH TO LEARNING

This book has been written for students and practicing radiographers to help them with the mathematical concepts that support the selections of technique factors. Likewise, this information is incorporated to encourage the student and radiographer to think in terms of an integrated system in the mathematics of exposure.

You will find that the more you work with and practice these problems and try to integrate the information into your daily practice of radiologic technology, the more proficient you will become at understanding and applying the principles of the mathematics of exposure.

Effective operation of radiographic equipment goes beyond learning the parts of the machine, the concepts of physics of x-ray production, accessories, anatomy, physiology, pathology.

In practice, the radiographer makes the independent decisions in positioning and selection of techniques, many of which are not to be found in technique charts or in textbooks.

Effective use of the radiographic exposure factors is key to helping the radiographer be successful in producing films of excellent diagnostic quality regardless of the situation.

STUDY TIPS

1. Study as soon as possible after class.

2. With mathematical problems, practice, practice, practice. Learn the long methods BEFORE you use any shortcuts.

3. Set up and do questions and practice problems.

4. Invest in an inexpensive calculator. The basic functions, add, subtract, multiply, divide, percent, and square root are sufficient for most problems.

5. If you get stuck or confused on how to do a problem, ask for help.

6. If one book does not have the answers to problems you can't solve, check other books. There are many good radiologic technology books available, and most libraries can obtain even the most obscure radiologic technology book.

7. Do not be afraid to make mistakes, but figure out how to make the corrections, too.

Pretest

The mathematical calculations used in radiographic exposure techniques are not a mystery as long as one remembers the following suggestions:

1. Know the rules for doing the calculations.

2. Know how to apply the rules accurately.

The explanations and problems in this book are presented with NO SHORTCUTS. The explanations are designed to help you understand "Why" certain rules are used and "How" the rules have been derived.

The problems in this teaching module have been written using exposure factors used in radiographic techniques.

To help you measure your progress, take the following pretest on ratios, proportions, and square root calculations. After completing this book you can compare your pretest and posttest results.

Directions

1. Answer each of the questions. Do not refer to any books or notes.

2. With each problem, write the formula for doing the calculation.

3. Do not use any shortcut methods.

4. When you finish, check your answers with the answer key on page 139. Make note of the incorrect answers, and use these as a guide for improving your skills.

If you have questions about the calculations, make a note of the questions. As you read and study this instructional workbook, many of your questions will be answered. If you still have questions, please see your instructor/tutor for additional explanations or write to me in care of the publisher.

1. A RATIO can also be called, in simplest terms:

    A. A fraction

    B. A term for an unknown number

    C. A square root

2. A RATIO defines:

    A. The difference between two numbers

    B. The equality of two numbers

    C. How many times larger *OR* smaller one number is to another.

3. In this ratio: $^{12}\!/_{24}$; the number on the bottom is the _____.

4. Convert the following numbers into ratios:

    A. 2″ is to 24″ = _____

    B. 15 is to 5 = _____

    C. 24 is to 12 = _____

5. A PROPORTION is a way of showing that two RATIOS are:

    A. Equal _____

    B. Unequal _____

6. How many factors are needed in a proportion to find an unknown number?

    A. One

    B. Two

    C. Three

7. Using the following formula, solve for "X" in the problem:

$$A : B :: C : D$$

A = 5; B = 10; C = "x"; D = 15
What is "X" equal to?

8. In the number "36^2", what does the "2" indicate?

   A. $36 \times 2 =$ _____

   B. $^{36}\!/_2 =$ _____

   C. $36 \times 36 =$ _____

9. What is a DIRECT PROPORTION? Please define.

10. What is an INVERSE PROPORTION? Define.

11. What is an INVERSE SQUARE LAW PROPORTION? Please define.

12. Define the term "Square Root."

13. What is the symbol for "Square Root?"

14. What is the "Square Root" of 3025?

15. Solve the following squared numbers:

   A. $36^2 =$ _____

   B. $40^2 =$ _____

   C. $55^2 =$ _____

   D. $72^2 =$ _____

   E. 103^2 cm = _____

After completing this PRETEST, check your answers against the key on page 139.

Parts of an Equation

Objectives

■ ■ ■ ■ ■ ■ ■ ■ ■ ■ ■

After studying this unit, the student should be able to:

1. Identify the parts of an equation.

2. Recall the parts of an equation.

3. Understand the relationship between the new and original factors in an equation.

4. Know the difference between superscript and subscript number and the functions of each.

5. Understand the function of a parenthesis in an equation.

   This unit will describe and explain the identification methods used in this book. This explanation will help you identify the specific parts of a formula so you will be able to set up the problems using the proper formula relationships. This information is vitally important. Memorize the parts of an equation. (See box on page 12.)

Parts of an Equation

- Original factors
- New factors
- Subscript numbers
- Superscript numbers (exponents)
- The unknown or "X" quantity

The following descriptions will help you know how the various factors in an equation are identified.

ORIGINAL FACTORS

These numbers, sometimes identified as the old factors, are the baseline upon which new techniques will be calculated.

The original factor placement in the formula will be identified through the use of lower case or small letters and the subscript number "1."

Example: i_1

NEW FACTORS

These factors indicate the changes to be used in the technique changes. These factors or numbers may also be the results of any changes made.

The new factor placement in the formula will be identified through the use of upper case or capital letters and the subscript number "2."

Example: I_2

SUBSCRIPT NUMBERS

Subscript numbers are numbers located at the LOWER RIGHT-HAND side of a number, and are used for identification only!

Example: mAs_1 or MAS_2

The previous examples show how lower case and capital letters combined with a subscript number can be used to identify the original and new parts of an equation. Both numbers "1" and "2" are subscript numbers because of their placement. These numbers also help you identify where the ORIGINAL and NEW factors are to be placed in the formula.

SUPERSCRIPT NUMBERS

These numbers are located at the UPPER RIGHT-HAND side of the number and have a specific use.

Example: Old factor with superscript: i^2
New factor with superscript: I^2

Superscript numbers are also called exponents. Superscript numbers or exponents indicate that the number is to be multiplied by itself a specific number of times. An exponent can be any quantity.

Example: 36^2 means 36×36
36^3 means $36 \times 36 \times 36$

So to summarize subscript and superscript numbers:

- The ORIGINAL SET OF FACTORS are designated by lower case or small letters with the subscript number "1."

- The NEW SET OF FACTORS are designated by upper case or capital letters and the subscript number "2."

- SUPERSCRIPT NUMBERS, also called exponents, indicate how many times a number is to be multiplied by itself.

Exponents, or superscript numbers, are used extensively in mathematics; however, in this book the discussion is limited to the basic applications in the mathematics of radiographic exposure, specifically distance applications.

If additional information on the use and various forms of exponents used in mathematical applications is desired, you should check other references that deal with this mathematical process. You will discover that exponents are a useful form of mathematical notation.

To summarize this discussion and exercise on exponents, recall:

1. An exponent, or superscript number, means the number of times a quantity is multiplied by itself. An exponent can be any amount, but regardless, the rules for the exponents do not change.

2. In reading numbers with an exponent, for example, 10^5, you would say, "Ten to the fifth power."

3. This means that 10 is multiplied by itself five times, or $10 \times 10 \times 10 \times 10 \times 10$. It does not mean: 5×10. It is imperative that you know this difference.

PARENTHESES

Parentheses ( ) indicate that a specific calculation should be done **BEFORE** other equation functions are performed.

As an example, review the following problem:

$$(2 \times 2) \div (8 - 3)$$

Before dividing, you will multiply $2 \times 2 = 4$. Then subtract 3 from $8 = 5$. Then divide 4 by 5, which is the last function. The answer is 0.8.

This symbol, $(\ )^2$, means that the number or numbers inside the parentheses are to be SQUARED.

For example: $(10)^2$ means $10 \times 10 = 100$. It also means: 10 to the second power or 10 squared.

If your numbers are $(5 \times 10)^2$, this means 5×10 squared or 50^2, which means $50 \times 50 = 2500$. The exponent outside the parentheses means that you will compute the product of the numbers inside the parentheses by itself the number of times specified by the exponent number.

If you have (5×10^2), first, multiply 10×10, as indicated. That is, 10^2, which is $10 \times 10 = 100$. Then multiply this product, 100, by 5, the other number in your problem. The result is 500.

If you get confused, review the rules for exponents and parentheses, and recalculate the problems.

Another parentheses/exponent form may look like this:

$$(10^5)$$

This notation means $10 \times 10 \times 10 \times 10 \times 10$, or 10 to the fifth power, and equals 100,000. This function of multiplication must be done before the other functions in the calculation are done.

You should be aware that other forms and uses of the exponent and the parentheses exist, but the forms explained in this book are an introduction to both the use of the parentheses and the exponent as they occur in doing the basic calculations in this book.

Before continuing, review the rules for doing the calculations on pages 12-14.

■ *Practice Problems*

For review and practice in using exponents and parentheses do these calculations and show the results.

You will recognize some of the numbers as distances commonly used in radiographic procedures.

1. 36^2 _____ × _____ = _____

2. 40^2 _____ × _____ = _____

3. 50^2 _____ × _____ = _____

4. 55^2 _____ × _____ = _____

5. 20^2 _____ × _____ = _____

6. 72^2 _____ × _____ = _____

7. 28^2 _____ × _____ = _____

8. 100^2 _____ × _____ = _____

9. $(50 - 10)^2$ _____ × _____ = _____

10. $(10^2) - 50$ _____ × _____ = _____

Check your answers against the key on page 139.

STUDY TIPS

Whenever you do a set of radiographic exposure problems, the following suggestions should help you. An example is included. Study the examples and use the suggested method. You will find that as you separate the components from the whole of the problem, it will be easier to see the relationship each part has to the whole and to the other parts of the problem.

These suggestions will help you memorize the correct formulas for the problems and help you better evaluate the various parts of the problem.

To facilitate your work on all the problems in this book, remember the following:

1. Read the problem completely.

    A. What are the known parts of the problem?

    B. Identify the unknown parts of the problem.

    C. What does the problem ask you to do?

2. Write the formula that you will be using.

3. Reread the problem and EXTRACT THE VITAL INFORMATION.

4. Write the correct formula as this example shows:

Formula Example:

$$\frac{mAs_1}{MAS_2} = \frac{d_1^2}{D_2^2}$$

Problem Example: In a specific technique, 10 mAs was used at 40″ SID. It was necessary to change the mAs to 5. What is the new distance?

PROCEDURE:

Step 1: Extract the vital information and write the numbers opposite the correct part of the formula.

$$mAs_1 = 10 \text{ ORIGINAL mAs}$$

$$MAS_2 = 5 \text{ NEW MAS}$$

$$d_1^2 = 40 \text{ ORIGINAL DISTANCE}$$

$$D_2^2 = \times \text{ UNKNOWN DISTANCE}$$

Step 2: Using the formula for solving mAs-Distance problems, REPLACE the letters in the formula with the numbers.

Step 3: Until you become used to identifying the parts of the problem easily, extract the vital information from the problem as shown in the above-described method.

Step 4: Do not use any shortcut methods until you are comfortable with the calculation procedure.

    Did you do the calculations for this problem? If not, give it a try. If you did, you are on the right track to success. The extra practice is useful.

■ Q U I Z

1. In this book, SUBSCRIPT numbers are used to identify:

   A. Unnecessary parts of a problem.

   B. Original factors of a problem.

   C. New factors of a problem.

   D. None of these.

   E. B and C.

2. SUBSCRIPT numbers are located:

   A. At the lower right-hand side of a number.

   B. At the upper right-hand side of a number.

3. SUPERSCRIPT numbers are located:

   A. At the upper left-hand side of a number.

   B. At the upper right-hand side of a number.

4. SUBSCRIPT numbers are used for identification purposes only.

   A. True

   B. False

5. SUPERSCRIPT numbers:

   A. Identify parts of an equation.

   B. Have no purpose.

   C. Indicate that a number is to be multiplied by itself a specific number of times.

   D. Indicate that a round-off error may occur.

6. Another name for a SUPERSCRIPT NUMBER is:

A. Divisor

B. Addend

C. Subtrahend

D. Exponent

See page 140 to check your answers.

Ratios

Objectives

■ ■ ■ ■ ■ ■ ■ ■ ■ ■ ■

Upon completion of this unit, you should be able to:

1. Define a RATIO and demonstrate this ability verbally or in writing.

2. Define a RATIO RELATIONSHIP and demonstrate this ability verbally or in writing.

3. Identify and label the parts of a RATIO.

4. Solve problems that require using the formula for ratios.

RATIOS are, in simplest terms, fractions that indicate the relationship of one number to another number, that is, how many times LARGER or SMALLER one number is to another.

A RATIO is written with a colon (:) between the two numbers or letters.

Example:

1. A:B
   This is read: "A" *is to* "B."

   This means $\frac{A}{B}$ -or- 'A" divided by "B."

2. 4:5, is the same as $\frac{4}{5}$

   which also means "4" divided by "5."

PARTS OF A RATIO

In a ratio, the number on top can be called the first term or the NUMERATOR.
The number on the bottom can be called the second term or the DENOMINATOR.

Example:

$$\frac{4 = \text{NUMERATOR}}{5 = \text{DENOMINATOR}}$$

WRITING A RATIO

To write a RATIO correctly, the following rules apply, and must be used:

RULE 1. Write the number asked about FIRST, the numerator, then write the number with which it is being compared, called the denominator.

RULE 2. Ratios are, in simplest terms, fractions, and indicate a DIVISION procedure.

Example: Student "A" took six chest radiographs, and student "B" took 24 chest radiographs. Student "B" took "X" times more radiographs than Student "A." What is "X" equal to?

Use a RATIO to solve and evaluate these numbers.

Procedure: Set up the ratio, with the number asked about in the numerator position as shown in this example:

$$\frac{24}{6} = 24 \text{ divided by } 6 = 4$$

Answer: Student "B" took four times more chest radiographs than Student "A."

If you want to report this information in the form of a fraction, you need to know total number of radiographs taken. So first, add the number of radiographs taken by both students: $24 + 6 = 30$ total number of radiographs.

Set up a fraction that answers this question: "X" is what part of the total?" Reduce to lowest terms.

Example:

$$6 \mid \frac{24}{30} = \frac{4}{5}$$

Answer: Student "B" took ⅘ of all the chest radiographs.

RULE 3:   The quantities compared in a ratio MUST be compared in the same units.

Example: Compare 12 inches to 4 feet.

Before setting up the RATIO, both numbers must be written in the same units: 12 inches = 1 foot; 4 feet = 48 inches. You may elect to use either feet, inches, or convert to the metric system.

IN INCHES: 12:48

IN FEET: 1:4

IN CENTIMETERS: (1 in = 2.54 cm; thus 12 inches = 30.48 cm)
therefore 48 inches = 121.92 cm

The resulting numbers, in centimeters, become:
30.48:121.92

IN METERS: 1 foot = 0.3048 meters
4 feet = 1.2192 meters becomes the ratio: 0.3048:1.2192

PRACTICAL APPLICATION OF RATIOS

Ratios are used to compare one technique, or one number, with another, and to make changes based on the resulting information.

In the next unit, technique changes for using grids with different ratios will be described.

Changing techniques from one grid ratio to another is easy, but you must know the conversion values of each grid as assigned by the manufacturer. Be sure you have this information.

You should memorize these methods and become familiar with making the necessary calculations.

To recap, RATIOS are the basis for understanding and using proportions that are commonly used in radiographic exposure technique calculations.

Remember: It is important to practice doing the calculations and mathematical manipulations to become proficient in working with the many technique conversions that may appear during the course of a radiographic procedure.

Using Ratios in Grid Changes

Hint: Become familiar with this technique change process, because you will use it with some frequency in this book as well as in day-to-day practice.

Converting a technique from one **grid ratio** to another is easy. Your objective will be to memorize and learn how to use these methods. Here is the formula for grid techniques that involve changes in grid ratios:

$$\text{New mAs} = \frac{\text{New Grid Factor}}{\text{Original Grid Factor}} \times \text{Original mAs}$$

This formula will give you a range in which to work with changes in grid ratios; however, you should be aware of the other factors that govern the amount of secondary radiation that is filtered out and the amount of primary radiation that actually reaches the film. Some useful references are Carlton-Adler, 1992; Cullinan-Cullinan, 1994; Hiss, 1993; Liebel-Flarsheim, 1987; Thompson, 1979.

Ratios and Radiographic Grids

One of the most common uses of the RATIO in radiography involves the use of grids.

Grids are used to decrease the adverse effects of scatter radiation that can interfere with obtaining a film of acceptable diagnostic quality.

Grids are classified in a variety of ways, but the most common classification is by **GRID RATIO.**

Grid Ratio: The height of the lead strips in the grid to the distance between the lead strips.

Grid Ratio is expressed by the following formula:

$$R = \frac{\text{H (Height of lead strips)}}{\text{D (Distance between lead strips)}}$$

For example: "If the height of the lead strips is 2.5 cm, and the distance between the strips is 0.5 cm, the **Grid Ratio is 5:1.**

We can verify this information by using the formula and the parameters given us:

$$\frac{\text{Height} = 2.5}{\text{Distance} = .5} = 5:1 \text{ ratio}$$

For more information, see Burns, 1993; Bushong, 1993; Carlton-Adler, 1992; Hiss, 1993; Leibel-Flarsheim, 1987; Meredith-Massey, 1977; Selman, 1985.

Changing Grids

Before one can change from one grid ratio to another, it is important to know the grid ratio conversion factors.

The following is a list of some commonly used grid conversion factors for grids with fiber interspacers. These factors will change under the following conditions: Number of lead strips/inch, kVp levels, type of interspace material used, and base technical factors within individual radiology departments.

Some useful references are Burns, 1993; Bushong, 1993; Carlton-Adler, 1993; Cullinan-Cullinan, 1994; Hiss, 1993.

With the improvement in manufacturing technology, the use of aluminum as an interspacer is more easily accomplished and efficient; thus grids with aluminum interspacers are more prevalent in the work place (Liebel-Flarsheim: 1987). Refer to the next section regarding how to obtain technical information about the grids you may be using.

The procedure for making technique conversions is an important part of becoming familiar with the mathematical rules that govern technique conversions.

The table below lists grid conversion factors based on relative exposure factors.

Grid Conversion Factors

Grid type	Factor
No grid	1
5:1	2
6:1	3
8:1	4
12:1	5
16:1	6

Note: Be sure to check with the grid manufacturer about conversion factors for specific grids.
Source: Thompson TT: Cahoon's formulating x-ray techniques, ed 9, Duke University Press, Durham NC, 1979.

Cross-Hatch Grids

Cross-hatch or criss-cross grids are those that have lead strips going in both directions across the grid. These grids have very specific uses; thus they are not often used in general radiographic practice. However, the student and radiographer should know about this type of grid and that, as with the linear grid, there are conversion factors for using these grids as well.

Cross-hatch grid factors:

5:1 = 5.5 at 85 kVp

8:1 = 7.5 at 85 kVp

(Liebel-Flarsheim, 1987)

Laminated Flexible Grid

Insight Thoracic Imaging

New technology such as the new grid that uses layers of lead sheets and as many as 27 million laser-aligned micro-holes rather than the conventional linear, parallel, or cross-hatch patterns, developed by Eastman Kodak, need not pose technical conversion problems for radiographers. Cullinan and Cullinan indicate that conversion factors for this grid are similar to those used for the standard 6:1 linear grid. This new grid will not have the focal distance constraints present in the conventional grid systems.

■ *Practice Problems*

As you recall, ratio problems are set up like fractions, and this ratio for changing grid ratios within a radiographic exposure technique is no different than any other ratio problem except that it has an additional step.

This step will be described in detail to help you learn how to manipulate the calculations properly.

The number written first, or numerator, is the number in question. This number is divided by the denominator. The resulting number is a conversion factor that you will use to adjust your radiographic technique.

For convenience in understanding this process, the following is how the two-step formula looks.

Step 1:

$$\frac{\text{New Grid Factor}}{\text{Original Grid Factor}} = \text{Conversion Factor}$$

Step 2: Conversion Factor × Original mAs = NEW mAs

You may have some other technique adjustments to make, but at this point, your only concern should be the proper uses of grids with different ratios and how you will deal with the technical factors.

Problem 1: Change from an **8:1 grid** to an **12:1** grid. 20 mAs was used with the 8:1 grid. What is the new mAs with a 12:1 grid?

PROCEDURE:

Step 1: What is the formula? Refer above if you don't remember.

Step 2: Write the equation using the numbers needed to do the problem.

           Grid ratios   Grid conversion factors

$$\frac{\text{12:1 (Grid changed to)}}{\text{8:1 (Original Grid)}} = \qquad \frac{5}{4} \qquad = 1.25$$

Step 3: Multiply the original mAs 20 × 1.25

ANSWER:

The new exposure for using the 12:1 grid is 25 mAs.

Problem 2: 60 mAs was used with a 16:1 grid. Change to a 5:1 grid. What is the new mAs?

PROCEDURE:

Step 1: What is the formula? If you've forgotten, refer to the previous section.

Step 2: Write the equation using the numbers needed.

$$\frac{5:1 \text{ (The new grid ratio factor)}}{16:1 \text{ (Original grid ratio factor)}} = \frac{2}{6} = .33$$

Step 3: Multiply 60 (your original mAs) × .33

ANSWER:

19.8 or 20 mAs

With an mAs that cannot be easily set on the machine, select the closest mAs. The slight differences in the mAs values are generally considered insignificant, assuming the kVp levels are proper for the part.

■ Q U I Z

1. What is a RATIO?

2. List two ways that a RATIO can be written using the values: A = 5; B = 10.

    1. _____   2. _____

3. In a RATIO, which number is written first?

4. What does a RATIO indicate about the numbers being compared?

5. When numbers are being compared in a RATIO, can inches be compared to centimeters? _____

6. How can two different units be compared?

PRACTICE WRITING THESE RATIOS:			
	With a colon	As a fraction	Lowest terms
7. 2″ is to 24″			
8. Team A won 5 out of 20 games			
9. 15 to 5			
10. 24 to 12			

	With a colon	As a fraction	Lowest terms
PRACTICE WRITING THESE RATIOS:			
11. 5:1 Grid = 2, 16:1 Grid = 6 Change 5:1 to 16:1 grid			
12. 1 ft is to 36″			
13. 10 min is to 1 hr			
14. 2 cm to 4 cm			
15. 8 cc to 20 cc			
16. 6 mR to 20 mR			

17. For a specific technique, 30 mAs was used with a 5:1 grid. It was desirable to use an 8:1 grid. What is the new mAs?

18. A 12:1 grid was used with 50 mAs. It was necessary to change to a 16:1 grid. What is the new mAs?

19. A technique of 10 mAs with an 8:1 grid was used. Change to a 16:1 grid. What is the new mAs?

20. Twenty mAs was used with a 16:1 grid, but a new technique required a change to a 6:1 grid. What is the new mAs?

Check your answers with the answer key on page 140. If you have several incorrect answers, review and practice the problems until your skills and score improve.

Proportions

Objectives

■ ■ ■ ■ ■ ■ ■ ■ ■ ■ ■

Upon completion of this unit, you should be able to:

1. Define numerical proportions and proportional relationships.

2. Write a proportion correctly.

3. Identify the parts of a proportion and label those parts correctly.

4. Solve for the unknown quantity in a proportion problem.

5. Correctly apply the mathematical rules that govern the calculations in proportional problems.

6. Check the calculations using the rules of mathematics.

A **PROPORTION** is a way of showing that two ratios are equal.

Example:

$$A:B = C:D$$

or

"A" is to "B" as "C" is to "D"

This proportion can be set up in the following way:

$$\frac{A}{B} = \frac{C}{D}$$

In these problems, the EQUAL sign (=) is read: "AS," and the DOT in a problem means MULTIPLY.

PARTS OF A PROPORTION

There are two parts of a proportion problem. These parts are the **EXTREMES** and the "MEANS."

In the examples listed above,

"A" and "D" are the EXTREMES.

"B" and "C" are the MEANS.

It is important to know the parts of a proportion, because it is an integral part of setting up the equation to be solved.

Also, knowing the parts of a proportion will be useful when you need to double-check the accuracy of your solution, because the product of the **MEANS** should equal the product of the **EXTREMES.**

In other words, the product of "A" × "D" should be the same as the product of "B" × "C."

PROPORTION RULES

Proportions are relatively simple to calculate IF you familiarize yourself with the rules that govern them.

PROPORTION RULE 1: As long as any three (3) factors in a proportion are known, the fourth or unknown factor can be found.

Example: In the following problem, solve for "X" by using this formula:

$$\frac{A}{B} = \frac{C}{D}$$

Problem:

$$A = 2; B = 4; C = \text{"x"}; D = 8$$

Procedure:

Step 1: Write the formula.

Step 2: Fill in the numerical values.

$$\frac{2}{4} = \frac{X}{8}$$

Step 3: MULTIPLY both sides of the equation by the number associated with "X."

$$8 \cdot \frac{2}{4} = \frac{X}{8} \cdot 8$$

Step 4: Cancel the "8"s on the "X" side of equation.

Step 5: Your equation should now look like this:

$$8 \cdot \frac{2}{4} = \frac{X}{\cancel{8}} \cdot \cancel{8}$$

Step 6: The "X" now stands alone, and your equation looks like this:

$$X = \frac{(8 \cdot 2)}{4}$$

Recall: The parentheses mean you must perform the indicated function before doing other functions; therefore 8 times 2 = 16, which is then divided by 4.

Your equation now looks like this: $X = \frac{16}{4}$

Step 7: Divide 16 by 4 to determine "X," the unknown quantity:

Answer: $X = 4$

Regardless of the position of the unknown quantity, or "X," in an equation, it is possible to find the solution. Look at the following examples and read the associated discussion. This will help you become comfortable with the procedures for dealing with the unknown, or "X," especially when it is in a denominator position.

These descriptions explain the procedures for the long method of problem calculations and are presented to help you understand as well as do the problems.

Do not use shortcut methods unless instructed to do so. As you gain experience, you will most likely use shortcut methods, but the experience must come first!

PROPORTION RULE 2: In a proportion, whenever you have an "X" or an unknown quantity in the numerator position and associated with a number, MULTIPLY both sides of the equation by that number.

Problem: A = 2; B = 4; C = X; D = 8

Procedure:

Step 1: Write the formula:

$$\frac{A}{B} = \frac{C}{D}$$

Step 2: Fill in the numerical values:

$$\frac{2}{4} = \frac{X}{8}$$

Step 3: Multiply BOTH sides of the equation by "8," which is the number associated with "X." Your equation should look like this:

$$8 \cdot \frac{2}{4} = \frac{X}{8} \cdot 8$$

Step 4: Cancel the numbers on the "X" side of the equation, which **LIBERATES** the "X" for easier calculation.

Step 5: Rewrite your equation. It should look like this:

$$X = \frac{8 \cdot 2}{4} = \frac{16}{4}$$

which is 16 divided by 4.

Answer: $X = 4$

PROPORTION RULE 3: Whatever is done to one side of the equation MUST be done to the other side of the equation.

PROPORTION RULE 4: Computing the equation is easier if the unknown quantity, or "X," is in the numerator position. Therefore whenever "X" is in the denominator position, **INVERT** that side of the equation so the "X" is on top or numerator position.

AND, the other side of the equation must also be inverted to maintain the proportional relationship.

Rule 3 and Rule 4 are similar in this way: BOTH sides of the equation MUST be treated equally.

In RULE 3 both sides of the equation can be multiplied by the number associated with "X," which liberates the "X." This does not change the numerical relationship.

This step is included to explain how equations are derived for streamlining the calculation. It is a useful way to learn how to do these calculations correctly.

And RULE 4 shows that by placing the unknown, or "X," in the numerator position, the calculations are more easily done.

Thus, in making the inversion on the "X" side of the equation, we must also INVERT the other side of the equation to maintain the numerical relationship in the proportion.

Example: In this example note that "X" is in the denominator position.

$$\frac{4}{2} = \frac{8}{X}$$

And because the calculations are much easier to do when "X" is in the numerator position, INVERT the equation, so the "X" becomes a numerator.

$$\frac{2}{4} = \frac{X}{8}$$

Remember: Whenever a proportion problem is set up for solution, the same values must be arranged in proper order.

In other words, like items must be placed with like items, for example, apples with apples and bananas with bananas. Study the following explanation for an in-depth look at this rule.

Example: Assume you have an original and a new mA and an original time and an unknown time in the problem statement.

Problem: The original mA was 100. The mA is to be changed to 500. The original time used was 0.5 seconds. What is your new time?

There are two options you can use in setting up a proportion problem. Closely examine the following examples and decide which option is easier for you to do.

Option One for proportion equation:

$$\frac{mA_1}{MA_2} = \frac{time_1}{TIME_2}$$

-OR-

Option Two for proportion equation.

$$\frac{mA_1}{time_1} = \frac{MA_2}{TIME_2}$$

Two relationships exist in these formulas.

The first relationship exists between the original and new mA values and the original and new time values. The second relationship exists between the ORIGINAL values mA and time, AND the relationship between NEW values of MA and TIME.

Notice how the formulas are structured to verify these statements, and understand these specific points in setting up a proportion equation, because it will make a difference in the accuracy of solving proportion problems.

REVIEW OF THE RULES

RULE 1: As long as any three (3) factors in a proportion are known, the fourth can be found.

RULE 2: Anytime you have "X" divided by a number, MULTIPLY both sides of the equation by that number.

RULE 3: Whatever is done to one side of the equation must also be done to the other side of the equation.

RULE 4: It is easier to compute the equation if the "X" is in the numerator position. Therefore INVERT the equation whenever "X" is a denominator.

RULE 5: Whenever a proportion problem is set up for solution, like values must be arranged in corresponding order.

Try the following practice problems. Refer to these rules if you need to do so.

■ *Practice Problems*

REMEMBER THIS FORMULA: A:B = C:D

Problem 1: A = 5; B = 10; C = X; D = 40

PROCEDURE:

Step 1: If the problem statement contains a lot of description, carefully read the problem and extract the vital information.

Step 2: Write the formula:

$$\frac{A}{B} = \frac{C}{D}$$

Step 3: Replace the letters in the formula with the numbers from the problem statement.

$$\frac{5}{10} = \frac{X}{40}$$

Step 4: Multiply BOTH sides of the equation by the number associated with "X."

$$40 \cdot \frac{5}{10} = \frac{X}{40} \cdot 40$$

Step 5: You can cancel the number "40" on the "X" side of the equation.

Step 6: Your equation should look like this:

$$X = 40 \cdot \frac{5}{10} = \frac{200}{10}$$

which is 200 divided by 10.

ANSWER:

     X = 20.

You will notice that by multiplying both sides of the equation by the number associated with "X," the "X" is liberated, which makes the equation easier to solve.

Try a problem that has the "X" in the denominator position.

RECALL the formula for proportions: A:B = C:D

Problem 2: A = 2; B = 4; C = 8; D = "X"

PROCEDURE:

Step 1: Carefully read the problem and extract the vital information.

Step 2: Write the formula:

$$\frac{A}{B} = \frac{C}{D}$$

Step 3: Replace the letters in the formula with the numbers from the problem statement.

$$\frac{2}{4} = \frac{8}{X}$$

Step 4: Invert BOTH sides of the equation so the "X" is in a numerator position.

$$\frac{4}{2} = \frac{X}{8}$$

Step 5: MULTIPLY BOTH SIDES of the equation by "8" to liberate the "X."

$$8 \cdot \frac{4}{2} = \frac{X}{8} \cdot 8$$

Step 6: Cancel where appropriate and complete the calculations.

ANSWER:

$$X = 16$$

Refer to this unit whenever you want to review the basic rules that govern how the calculations for proportions should be done.

REMEMBER: Do not use any shortcut calculation methods unless you are instructed to do so. You will have plenty of time to develop the shortcuts after you have mastered the methods that will help you learn both "how and why" a problem is solved.

1. A = 6; B = 25; C = X; D = 35

2. A = 8; B = 64^2; C = 40; D = X^2

3. 18:9 :: X:6

4. A = 10^3; B = X; C = 25^3; D = 50

5. A = 16; B = 4; C = 15; D = X

6. X:12 :: 20:50

Check your answers with the answer key on page 141.

Direct, Inverse, and Inverse-Square Proportions

Objectives

■ ■ ■ ■ ■ ■ ■ ■ ■ ■ ■

Upon completion of this unit, you should be able to:

1. Differentiate between DIRECT, INVERSE, and INVERSE SQUARED PROPORTIONS, and be able to demonstrate this knowledge in writing or verbally.

2. Do the calculations that involve solving for an unknown quantity in a DIRECT, INVERSE, or INVERSE SQUARE PROPORTIONAL PROBLEM.

3. Identify and label the parts of a proportional problem.

DIRECT PROPORTIONS

A **DIRECT PROPORTION** is one in which one quantity maintains the same ratio to a quantity as the latter changes. FOR EXAMPLE: A:B, and IF "B" is doubled, "A" is automatically DOUBLED.

Example: **DIRECT PROPORTION FORMULA**

$$\frac{a_1}{b_1} = \frac{A_2}{B_2}$$

Compare these two similar triangles:

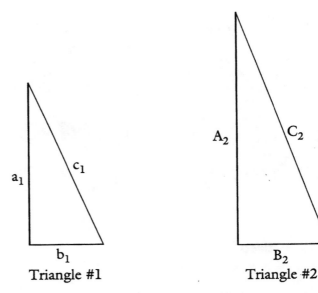

Triangle #1   Triangle #2

In this example, if side (C_1) of Triangle 1 is increased as shown in Triangle 2, the corresponding sides of Triangle 2, A_2 and B_2, will be proportionately increased. These triangles with the corresponding changes show a **DIRECT PROPORTION** relationship.

Direct Proportions Commonly Used in Radiography

1. **TIME and DISTANCE^2:**

$$\frac{t_1}{T_2} = \frac{d_1^2}{D_2^2}$$

2. **MILLIAMPS-SECONDS and DISTANCE^2 (with constant time.)**

$$\frac{mAs_1}{MAS_2} = \frac{d_1^2}{D_2^2}$$

3. **MILLIAMPS and DISTANCE^2:**

$$\frac{mA_1}{MA_2} = \frac{d_1^2}{D_2^2}$$

Review these formulas and study the **Direct Relationship** until you can recall them without referring to the textbook.

Remember: In a direct proportion problem, the relationships in Time, Distance, Milliamps, sizes, and shapes will increase or decrease proportionately to the amount of increase or decrease in distance.

■ *Practice Problems*

In a *Direct Proportion*, the factors are **directly** proportional to each other.

MAS and distance are **directly proportional.** Study the formula that supports this directly proportional relationship.

Direct Proportion formula: mAs and Distance

$$\frac{mAs_1}{MAS_2} = \frac{d_1^2}{D_2^2}$$

Problem 1: The technique was 50 mAs at 40″ SID. We changed the distance to 72″ SID. What mAs is needed to maintain the original levels of density on the film?

PROCEDURE:

Step 1: Write the formula to be used.

$$\frac{mAs_1}{MAS_2} = \frac{d_1^2}{D_2^2}$$

Step 2: Extract the vital information from the problem and label accordingly.

$$mAs_1 = 50$$

$$MAS_2 = \text{``X''}$$

$$d_1^2 = 40^2$$

$$D_2^2 = 72^2$$

Step 3: Replace the letters in the formula with the numbers from the problem. The equation should look like this:

$$\frac{50}{X} = \frac{40^2}{72^2}$$

Step 4: REMEMBER: "X" should be in the numerator position, so when you invert the left-hand side of the equation to make this change, you MUST also invert the right hand side of the equation.

$$\frac{X}{50} = \frac{72^2}{40^2}$$

Multiply both sides of the equation by the number associated with "X," and cancel. This "liberates" the "X" for easier calculation. Your equation should look like this:

$$\cancel{50} \cdot \frac{X}{\cancel{50}} = \frac{72^2}{40^2} \cdot 50$$

Step 5: After cancelling the appropriate numbers, the equation should look like this:

$$X = \frac{(72^2)50}{40^2} \quad \text{-OR-} \quad X = \frac{(72 \times 72)50}{40 \times 40}$$

Step 6:

$$X = \frac{259200}{1600}$$

ANSWER:

X = 162 mAs.

We have determined that 162 mAs at 72" SID is needed to obtain a film that will have a density level comparable to the original film taken at 40" SID.

In the following segment, three more problems are provided. Show all phases of your calculations. Do not use any shortcut methods unless instructed to do so.

Problem 2: A specific technique was 20 mAs at 36" SID. The distance was changed to 50" SID. What is the new mAs?

Problem 3: With a constant mA, the distance used for a technique was 40″ SID with an exposure time of 0.2 second. The distance is changed to 60″ SID. What is the new time? (Time: The length of exposure; a unit, expressed in seconds or fractions thereof, or combined as milliamps-seconds, during which time x-rays are produced.)

Problem 4: The mA was 200 at a distance of 72″ SID. The time was constant, but the distance was changed to 36″ SID. What is the new MA?

Once you have completed these problems, see page 141 and check your answers. Evaluating any problem areas you may have in making the calculations and review as needed. Take the quiz to check what you have learned thus far about proportions.

1. What is a direct proportion?

2. What happens when one side of the equation is doubled?

3. What are three commonly used direct proportion equations used in radiography?

4. What are the subscript numbers used for?

5. What are the superscript numbers used for?

6. If you should see a number written like this, 36^2, what does it mean? How would you make the calculation? What is the answer? _____.

7. What are the two ways that a Ratio or Direct Proportion can be written?

8. In this book both small and CAPITAL letters are used in the formulas. Of what use are these indicators in helping you identify the component part of the formula?

See page 142 to check your answers.

A METHOD FOR CHECKING CALCULATIONS

As we have discussed, proportional problems are also **RATIOS.** The solutions to proportion problems can be checked in an easy method. Here is how it works:

RATIOS have two main parts:

The extremes

The means

A ratio is often written like this: $A:B = C:D$.

"A" and "D" are the **EXTREMES.**

"B" and "C" are the **MEANS.**

To check the calculations we need only know that:

"The product of the EXTREMES should be equal or nearly equal to the product of the MEANS." The phrase "nearly equal" means there may be a **slight** difference in the results due to round-off error.)

Equal Example: $A:B = C:D$

$$1:2 = 2:4$$

Procedure:

Step 1:   MULTIPLY THE Extremes: $A \times D$

$$1 \times 4 = 4$$

Step 2:   MULTIPLY THE Means: $B \times C$

$$2 \times 2 = 4$$

Answer: Because the Extremes = 4 and the Means = 4, we can be assured that our problem has been correctly solved. If the results are nearly equal, as in the following example, you may have round-off error.

Nearly Equal Example:

$$A:B = C:D$$

$$7:27 = 3.88:15$$

Procedure:

Step 1.   Multiply the "Extremes" in the formula.

$$A \times D$$

$$7 \times 15 = 105$$

Step 2. Multiply the "Means."

$$B \times C$$

$$27 \times 3.88 = 104.76 \text{ or } 105$$

or

Rounding off numbers and its effect on checking these calculations:

You can round-off 3.88 to 3.9; multiply 3.9 by 27, which equals 105.3. Both numbers are close enough to the product of the Extremes that you can safely say that calculations are correct.

If the problem is set up incorrectly, the differences will be very obvious. Also, if incorrect answers have been obtained, the difference will indicate that the problem should be recalculated.

This is a useful method for checking your calculations as well as for doing the problems. It is helpful to be familiar with the procedure.

Review and practice the following problem until you are familiar with the calculation procedures.

Example:

$$mAs_1 : MAS_2 = d_1^2 : D_2^2$$

$$50 : 162 = 40^2 : 72^2$$

Step 1: Multiply the **EXTREMES**

$$mAs_1 \times D_2^2$$

$$50 \times (72 \times 72) = 259200$$

Step 2: Multiply the **MEANS**

$$MAS_2 \times d_1^2$$

$$162 \times (40 \times 40) = 259200$$

STUDY TIPS

When studying mathematical problems, it helps to design some problems yourself. When you design your own set of problems, especially if you are still learning how to do the calculations, the following hints will help.

Use one of the problems that you've done as a pattern to set up your "designer" problem. Just insert new numbers with which to work.

When you have completed the calculations on the self-designed problem, proceed to the next steps to verify and check your answers.

Working with exposure problems should be fun as well as challenging. You will see how both fun and challenges emerge from knowing how to do these problems when you evaluate the resultant radiographic films.

The films that result from any technique change will provide you with the opportunity to evaluate whether your technique selections have been proper. Check with your instructors regarding teaching films.

Words of Caution: Patients should **never** be used in "experimental" exposure technique changes.

Until you have gained both experience and skill in assessing the resultant films, all experimentation with changing exposure technique values should be done using a phantom or a step-wedge.

When you have gained experience in working with changing exposure factors, you may be faced with making these changes during the course of an actual procedure.

COMMONLY USED INVERSE PROPORTIONS

In an INVERSE PROPORTION, as one quantity varies, the other quantity varies in the OPPOSITE direction.

Stated another way: As one quantity increases, the other quantity decreases and vice-versa.

As an example, let's consider the action of a see-saw:

When the see-saw is balanced, distance A-B is proportional to distance C-D.

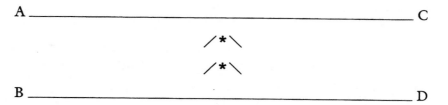

But when we decrease the distance A-B, the distance C-D is increased.

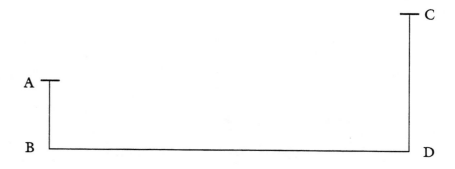

When we decrease distance C-D, the distance A-B is increased.

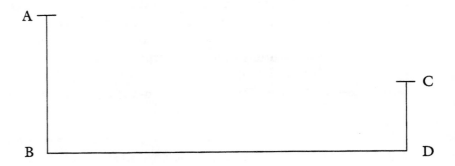

This example illustrates that as one quantity is decreased the other is increased, and it is this concept that exists in the inverse proportional relationships in dealing with x-rays and light. The following formulas are inversely proportional. Study them closely, because you will work with them on a daily basis.

Milliamps and (Exposure) Time

$$\frac{mA_1}{MA_2} = \frac{TIME_2}{time_1}$$

Intensity and Distance

This is the Inverse Square Law Formula. (Intensity, the rate of flow of roentgens, or energy)/unit of time.)

$$\frac{i_1}{I_2} = \frac{D_2^2}{d_1^2}$$

This formula, though **INVERSE** in its relationship, includes **squared** distances. Because of this special distance aspect, it will be discussed in a specific segment in this book.

■ Q U I Z

1. What is an inverse proportion?

2. List two radiographic formulas that are inverse in their relationship.

   1. _____

   2. _____

3. In an inverse proportion,

   A. When one quantity in the equation increases, the other quantity

   _____.

   B. When one quantity in the equation decreases, the other quantity

   _____.

4. In a certain procedure, the technique used was: 10 mA at 1 second. Because of motion, it was desirable to change the mA to 100. What is the new exposure time?

5. The following technique was used for an exam: 0.1 (1/10) second at 500 mA. The exposure time was changed to .05 seconds. What is the new mA?

When you have completed this unit test, check your answers against the answer key on page 142. If you are having problems doing these calculations, review the unit and set up some practice problems for yourself. Do not go to the next unit until you are able to do these problems easily.

MILLIAMPS AND EXPOSURE TIME

Milliamps and exposure time are inversely proportional. As the mA is increased, the exposure time is decreased. Likewise, as the time is increased, the mA is decreased.

The formula for Milliamps and Exposure Time is:

$$\frac{mA_1}{MA_2} = \frac{T_2}{t_1}$$

or

$$\frac{mA_2}{mA_1} = \frac{t_1}{T_2}$$

These two formulas are, in fact, the same, but have been presented to show you that in writing the formula, the inverse relationship must be maintained for the problem to work properly in the inverse relationship. This formula supports the main idea that when the milliamperage is increased, the exposure time can be decreased.

These problems are calculated using the same procedure used for the INVERSE PROPORTION problems, but notice there are no squared factors.

■ *Practice Problem*

Problem. The mA used is 200 and the exposure time is .1 second. The exposure time is changed to 0.05 second. What is the new mA?

PROCEDURE:

Step 1: Write the formula:

$$\frac{mA_1}{MA_2} = \frac{T_2}{t_1}$$

Step 2: Extract the vital information from the problem and write it down:

$$mA_1: 200$$

$$MA_2: X$$

$$t_1: 0.1$$

$$T_2: 0.05$$

Step 3: Set up the equation, replacing the letters with the numbers from the problem.

$$\frac{200}{X} = \frac{.05}{.1}$$

Step 4: "X" should be in the numerator position, so invert that side of the equation and the other side as well.

$$\frac{X}{200} = \frac{.1}{.05}$$

Step 5: Multiply both sides of the equation by the number associated with "X." This will liberate the "X" for easier calculation. Your equation should look like this:

$$\cancel{200} \cdot \frac{X}{\cancel{200}} = \frac{.1}{.05} \cdot 200$$

Cancel the 200 on the "x" side of the equation, which will liberate the "X."

Step 6: Your equation now looks like this:

$$X = \frac{.1 \cdot 200}{.05} = \frac{20}{.05}$$

$$X = 400 \text{ MA}$$

WATCH YOUR DECIMAL PLACEMENT!

Do the following problems using the INVERSE PROPORTION method.

1. The mA used was 500 and the exposure time was .05 second. Your mA was changed to 1000. What is the new exposure time?

2. The exposure time used was .5 second at 100 mA. You changed your exposure time to .25. What is the new mA?

3. The exposure time used was .005 at 600 mA. You changed your exposure time to .01. What is your new mA?

4. The milliamperage used for a technique is 300 and the exposure time is 0.3 seconds. You wish to use 900 mA. From this information, calculate the following:

   A. The ORIGINAL mAs = _____

   B. The NEW exposure time = _____

   C. The NEW mAs = _____

   D. Is the NEW mAs value the same or different from the ORIGINAL mAs value?

   Answer: _____

5. You use .5 second at 10 mA (5 mAs), but decide that the milliamperage is too low.

   Increase your milliamperage 10 times and adjust the exposure time accordingly.

   What is your new mA? _____

   What is your new exposure time? _____

   What is your new mAs? _____

Check your answers on page 142.

INVERSE SQUARE PROPORTIONS

Inverse Square Proportions are commonly used in radiographic techniques. This proportion, called the INVERSE SQUARE LAW (ISL), is special because it is key in understanding how both x-rays and light react when distance is changed, although our discussion will be limited to x-rays.

In addition to the inverse proportionate relationship, it is imperative to remember that distances in an ISL are squared.

Inverse Square Law

The intensity of the x-ray beam is inversely proportional to the square of the distance.

Our **OBJECTIVE** in this section is that you will be able to discuss and work with Inverse Square proportion problems.

The law is easily memorized, but learning the formula and the concepts behind it are vitally important.

Inverse Square Law Formula:

$$\frac{I_2}{i_1} = \frac{d_1^2}{D_2^2}$$

The Inverse Square Law can be written in another way, but for now, it is enough to become familiar with both the definition and one way to write this important radiological fact.

Recall that squared numbers are indicated by the superscript numbers that indicate how many times a number is multiplied by itself. When you are solving an ISL problem, you must remember that distances are **ALWAYS** squared; thus the final solution to an X^2 requires that you find its square root.

While this unit contains the basic information for finding the square root of a number without a calculator, the availability of small hand calculators makes this computation easier as you work through this book.

Also, you will find that most distances used in radiographic procedures are generally constant, which makes it easier to remember the square roots of most common Source-Image-Distances. However, it is advisable that you familiarize yourself with the procedure for doing the calculations without a calculator so you understand how the concept of square root governs an important aspect of the radiological application of the Inverse Square Law.

Before doing any of the calculations associated with the Inverse Square Law, try the following simple experiment.

A Simple Experiment

Objective: To demonstrate the effect of distance changes on the **INTENSITY** of the light (x-ray) beam.

After this experiment, you should be able to:

1. Discuss the application of the Inverse Square Law as it relates to x-rays and light.

2. Discuss the formula for the Inverse Square Law.

Practical experiments are useful in helping us to understand how principles and rules apply to our daily work as radiographers.

Do this experiment before continuing with the in-depth discussion on the Inverse Square Law. It is designed to demonstrate what happens in the Distance-X-ray Beam intensity relationship in radiography as well as give you a strong introduction to inverse proportional relationship.

This experiment is an adaptation of practical experiments discussed in *Thompson's Formulating X-Ray Techniques,* 9th Edition.

Materials:

1. A light source such as a flashlight that has new batteries and fresh light bulb. This experiment will not demonstrate the effects of distance on the intensity of the light unless these conditions are met.

2. A measuring stick.

3. A light-colored surface.

4. A semi-darkened room.

5. A light meter (optional).

Procedure:

1. Position your light source and mark the spot.

2. From this fixed location, MEASURE AND MARK two distances from a fixed large, light-colored surface: (a) 36 inches and (b) 72 inches.
   Note: This experiment can be done using an x-ray source, film, pocket dosimeter or light meter, or distances in the metric system. If films are to be exposed, phantoms should be used.

3. Position the light source at 36 inches from a light-colored surface.

4. Turn on the light source.

5. Visually, or with a light meter, (a) make note of the intensity or brightness of the lighted area, and (b) using a small piece of tape and paper, mark the outer perimeter of the circle of light, plus the vertical and horizontal intersection of the diameter of the circle.

This concludes the first part of the experiment, and now you will need to do the second part so you can see how changing distance from 36 inches to 72 inches affects the brightness of the light and the size of the lighted area.

For the second half of this experiment, turn off the light source, move the light source to the 72 inches mark, and turn on the light source.

As with the first part of this experiment, visually, or with a light meter, make (c) note of the brightness of the lighted area at 72 inches and the size of the lighted area, and (e) with a small piece of tape and paper, mark the outer perimeter of the circle of light, plus the vertical and horizontal intersection of the diameter.

If doing visual comparisons rather than using a light meter, two light sources should be used simultaneously and side by side. Set one at 36 inches and the other at 72 inches.

Here are some questions related to the experiment to think about and discuss.

1. Is there a noticeable difference between the intensity or brightness of the slight at 36 inches and at 72 inches?

2. At which distance is the intensity or brightness of the lighted area:

   MORE INTENSE _____

   LESS INTENSE _____

3. Is there a difference in the size of the circles of light?

4. Why is there a difference in brightness? Explain in your own words. What is your rationale for your explanation?

5. What is the name of the law that governs this change in brightness or intensity?

6. What other facts, historical or scientific, do you find significant about how this law works for or against the production of radiographs?

When you have completed the experiment and the discussion questions, continue to the next section.

You've come a long way in learning many of the details involved in working with mathematics of radiographic exposure. Your understanding of these many details will become easier as you gain experience. Remember the following:

> The Inverse Square Law is an inversely proportional relationship

IMPACT OF THE INVERSE SQUARE LAW

The Inverse Square Law states: **The intensity of the x-ray beam varies inversely with the square of the distance.** What does this mean? It means, very simply, that the intensity or the concentration of energy in the x-ray beam will change when the distance changes.

More specifically, if the distance is increased, the intensity, or concentration of energy, will decrease. If the distance is decreased, the intensity will increase. Subsequent to this change in the intensity is the manner in which the recorded image on the film is affected.

The word **intensity** describes the **general characteristics** of the beam of radiation as it is emitted from the x-ray tube and its concentration of energy and power in a specified area for a specific time. Intensity is simply a general word that encompasses many specific aspects and characteristics of the x-ray beam.

The description is a lot to think about at one time, but remember it is a term used to describe the beam of radiation from a general viewpoint, or "the big picture."

If you wish to examine the specific components that make up the intensity of the beam of x-radiation, refer to the recommended reading list and the bibliography. To discuss intensity fully in this text would detract from the purpose of this book.

But there are some specific points about intensity of the x-ray beam as it relates to the Inverse Square Law (ISL) that radiographers must learn to use. These points are key elements in understanding how the ISL affects the production and diagnostic quality of the recorded image.

The primary consideration is distance. If distance is doubled, the intensity of the x-ray beam is decreased four (4) times, or by one fourth of its original intensity.

For example, if two radiographs, one taken at 36″ SID and one at 72″ SID, **without** a compensatory change in the technique factors are compared, you will find that the film exposed at 72″ SID will be four times lighter than the film exposed at 36″ SID.

Conversely, if a film is exposed with a proper technique at 72″ SID, and the distance is decreased to 36″ SID **without** change in the technique factors, the intensity of the x-ray beam is increased four (4) times its original intensity. The film exposed at 36″ SID will be four (4) times darker than the film exposed at 72″ SID.

If changes are made in Source-Image-Distance, the radiographic exposure technique factors must be adjusted accordingly and in the proper proportion to the needs dictated by the SID change.

If you have difficulty understanding the ISL, repeat the experiment that demonstrates the principles of the Inverse Square Law.

If you want to actually see the changes in the density levels on a radiograph when distances are doubled or halved, use an aluminum step wedge to make the exposures. Ask your instructor for assistance.

The Inverse Square Law is expressed as an inversely proportionate ratio. The formula looks like this:

$$\frac{I_2}{i_1} = \frac{d_1^2}{D_2^2}$$

The formula might also be written like this:

$$\frac{i_1}{I_2} = \frac{D_2^2}{d_1^2}$$

In many of the reference books, you will see the ISL formula written both ways. Both methods are correct as long as the inverse proportionate relationship is maintained.

Recall: The subscript numbers indicate original (1) factor and new (2) factor. Superscript numbers or exponents indicate a specific mathematical procedure that must be done to correctly solve the problem.

The INVERSE SQUARE LAW effectively defines the results of any change in distance on the intensity of the X-ray beam. This law also holds true with respect to visible light.

As a radiographer, it is imperative that you commit the ISL, its concepts, formula, and effects to memory. It is your responsibility to make the exposure adjustments that will result in the proper density-contrast relationship of the finished radiograph when the distance is changed, assuming that the initial exposure factors are correct.

To check your understanding of the ISL discussion so far, complete the following quiz.

1. What is the definition of the Inverse Square Law?

2. Write the formula for the Inverse Square Law.

3. If the ISL can be written another way, please write it.

4. How does the Inverse Square Law work in radiography?

5. What happens to the intensity of the x-ray beam when the distance is:

   A. Doubled: _____

   B. Halved: _____

6. If you must solve for the distance in an Inverse Square Law Proportion, what additional information is needed once you have solved X^2?

Check your answers on page 143 in the answer key, and proceed to the next segment.

   If you have incorrectly answered any of the questions, review the previous section.

Remember the following:

> When calculating problems that involve the Inverse Square Law, distance changes require special attention and additional calculations BECAUSE both the known and the unknown distances are squared.

■ *Practice Problems*

A simple hand calculator that has the square root function will be most helpful in working these problems.

Problem 1: The new intensity of the x-ray beam is found to be 4 mR/min at 72″ SID. The original distance was 36″ SID. What was the original intensity of the x-ray beam?

PROCEDURE:

Step 1: Write the formula:

$$\frac{I_2}{i_1} = \frac{d_1^2}{D_2^2}$$

Step 2: Extract the vital information from the problem and write it in a vertical column.

$$I_2 = 4 \text{ mR/min}$$
$$i_1 = \text{``X''}$$
$$D_2^2 = 72^2$$
$$d_1^2 = 36^2$$

Step 3: Set up the equation using the numbers given in place of the letters in the formula:

$$\frac{4}{X} = \frac{36^2}{72^2}$$

Step 4: Because the "X" is in the denominator position, you MUST invert the equation so the "X" becomes a numerator.

$$\frac{X}{4} = \frac{72^2}{36^2}$$

Step 5: Multiply both sides of the equation by 4 (the number associated with "X") so that "X" will be liberated. Your equation now looks like this:

$$\cancel{4} \cdot \frac{X}{\cancel{4}} = \frac{72^2}{36^2} \cdot 4$$

Cancel the 4s on the "X" side of the equation.

Step 6: Your equation should now look like this:

$$X = \frac{72^2 \times 4}{36^2}$$

$$X = \frac{(72 \times 72)4 = 20736}{(36 \times 36) = 1296}$$

ANSWER:

$$X = 16 \text{ mR/min}$$

Note that the problems that follow involve DISTANCE changes.

Problem 2: A distance of 72″ SID and 10 mR was used. The mR is to be changed to 20 mR. What distance is needed?

PROCEDURE

Step 1: Write the formula:

$$\frac{I_2}{i_1} = \frac{d_1^2}{D_2^2}$$

Step 2: Extract the vital information from the problem and write it in a vertical column.

$$I_2 = 20 \text{ mR}$$

$$i_1 = 10 \text{ mR}$$

$$d_1^2 = 72^2$$

$$D_2^2 = X^2$$

Step 3: Set up the equation using the numbers given in place of the letters in the formula:

$$\frac{20}{10} = \frac{72^2}{X^2}$$

Step 4: Invert both sides of the equation so that "X^2" becomes a numerator:

$$\frac{10}{20} = \frac{X^2}{72^2}$$

Step 5: Liberate the "X^2."

$$72^2 \cdot \frac{10}{20} = \frac{X^2}{\cancel{72^2}} \cdot \cancel{72^2}$$

As you have previously done, cancel the two numbers associated with the "X." This will liberate the "X" for easier calculation. REWRITE your equation to look like this:

$$X^2 = \frac{(72 \times 72)10}{20} = 2592$$

$$X^2 = 2592$$

Step 6: Find the square root of 2592. Using a hand calculator is the easiest way to figure this out.

ANSWER:

50.9″ SID or 51″ SID, your new distance.

Whenever we need to find a new distance in a radiographic Inverse Square Proportion technique problem, the last step in the calculation will require that you find the square root of X^2.

Now try the next four practice problems on your own.

GOOD LUCK!

Note: The term *exposure rate* incorporates two ideas: radiation exposure and unit of time, thus resulting in an amount of radiation per a specific unit of time.

Problem 3: The exposure rate at 40″ SID is 30 mR/min. What is the exposure rate at 20″ SID?

■ ***Problem 4:*** The exposure rate at 36″ SID is 10 mR/min. What is the exposure rate at 72″ SID?

■ ***Problem 5:*** The exposure rate at 72″ SID is 2.5 mR/min. What is the exposure rate at 36″ SID?

Problem 6: The intensity of the x-ray beam at 20″ SID is 120 mR/min. What is the exposure rate at 40″ SID?

See page 143 in the answer key to check your answers. Evaluate your progress. Remember you can always review the rules and steps in solving these problems.

The next four problems will help you polish your skills in another area of the Inverse Square proportions: FINDING DISTANCE.

Remember:

1. Distances are squared.

2. You will need to find the square root of the unknown.

Problem 7: The exposure rate at 40″ SID is 30 mR/min. Change the exposure rate to 120 mR/min. What distance is needed?

Problem 8: The exposure rate at 36″ SID is 10 mR/min. What distance is needed to change the exposure rate to 2.5 mR/min?

Problem 9: The exposure rate at 72″ SID is 2.5 mR/min. The exposure rate is changed to 10 mR/min. What distance is needed?

Problem 10: At 20″ SID, an exposure rate of 120 mR/min is used. To obtain 60 mR/min, what new SID is needed?

Check your answers against the answers on page 143 sheet. If you are still having difficulty with these calculations, review and practice the unit on Inverse Square Law problems, both with unknown intensity and with distance, until you have mastered the procedures.

Remember: To fully understand how the Inverse Square Law works in radiology, you must understand the relevance of squared numbers and how to find the square root of a number.

FINDING SQUARE ROOTS WITHOUT A CALCULATOR

The availability of inexpensive, hand-held calculators has made the computation of square roots very simple. However, it is useful to be familiar with the procedure whether or not you have a calculator.

The procedure is easy to do, and it will help you understand the process behind the often misunderstood square root process.

Note: that in radiology, the use of square roots is most often associated with Inverse Square Law proportion problems. You should commit to memory the square roots of the most commonly used distances in radiology:

a) 36″   b) 40″   c) 72″

Do you commonly work in the metric system? If so, these numbers become:

(a) 81.4 cm;   (b) 101.6; (102) cm;   (c) 175.88 (176) cm

Practice Problems

■

Problem 1: What is the square root of 1038?

PROCEDURE:

Step 1: Set up your problem:

$$\sqrt{10.38}$$

Step 2: Mark two decimal places from the right-hand number. In this case that number is 8, and the decimal will go between the "0" and the "3."

Step 3: Ask yourself, "What number, when multiplied times itself, is equal to, or less than, the first two digits?"

For example: $2 \times 2 = 4$; $3 \times 3 = 9$; $4 \times 4 = 16$; and so forth. The logical number would be 3.

Step 4: Place that number on the left-hand side of the square root sign and above the second number of the first two numbers.

Step 5: Multiply the two numbers and place the product below the 10 and subtract. Then bring down the next two numbers.

$$
\begin{array}{r}
3 \\
3 \sqrt{10 \ . \ 38} \\
\underline{| \ 9 } \\
1 \ \ \ 38
\end{array}
$$

Step 6: To find the next divisor, ADD the first divisor to the multiplier. The next divisor becomes "6."

$$
\begin{array}{r}
3 \ \ \ \ 2. \\
3 \sqrt{10. \ \ 38. \ \ 00} \\
+3 \ | \ 9 \\
\hline
6 \ \ \ 1 \ \ \ 38
\end{array}
$$

$\rightarrow$

Step 7: Another number is needed to arrive at a number large enough to be equal to or less than 138.

Step 8: Let's try "2" and place at right side of 6. Multiply this number, 62, by 2, the divisor. $62 \times 2 = 124$.

Step 9: Place the 2 above the "8" in the last two numbers of the number to be solved.

Step 10: Bring 124 down and subtract it from 138.

$$
\begin{array}{r}
3 \quad\ 2. \\
3\ \overline{\smash{)}10.\ \ 38.00} \\
+3\ |\ \ 9 \\
\hline
138 \\
62\ |\ \ 124 \\
+\ 2 \\
\hline
64\quad\ 1400 \\
\end{array}
$$

Step 11: Add a decimal point and add two zeros. Bring the two zeros down to 14, which becomes 1400.

Step 12: Add 2 to 62 = 64. Then determine your next divisor/multiplier. Try 2. ($642 \times 2 = 1284.$) **Two** is the divisor/multiplier we need. You can continue to solve this problem.

Answer:

The complete answer is 32.218007, but one or two decimal points is usually sufficient.

You can check your calculations by multiplying the answer by itself and adding any remainders to the answer.

Problem 2: Suppose you have an uneven grouping of numbers that need square root calculations, for example: 10380

Procedure:

Step 1: Beginning at the right-hand side of your unknown number, 10380, mark off two decimal places throughout the entire number set.

Step 2: Your number should look like this: **1. 03. 80.**

Step 3: Select a number that when multiplied by itself is equal to or less than the first number to be divided. Multiply those numbers and place the product below the number being considered, as demonstrated in the example.

$$
\begin{array}{r}
1 \\
1\ \overline{\smash{)}1.\ \ 03.\ \ 80} \\
1 \\
\hline
03 \\
\end{array}
$$

Step 4: Consider the next set of numbers, "03." What number can be selected for the divisor? The answer is "2." Are there any numbers that when multiplied by themselves will equal "03?" The number selected for the divisor is "0."

$$
\begin{array}{r}
1 \phantom{\sqrt{1.\ 03.\ 80}} \\
1 \ \overline{\sqrt{1.\ 03.\ 80}} \\
+\underline{1 \ \ 1} \\
20 \mid \ \ 03 \ \ 80
\end{array}
$$

Continue the calculations to complete the problem.

Step 5: The process of finding a divisor is the same as used for even numbers. This square root will contain numbers after the decimal, so proceed until you have found the solution to the problem.

ANSWER:

101.88.

As you can see in square root calculations, the addition of a zero can vastly change the answer of a number.

1. At 36″ SID, the mR was 5. The mR was changed to 1.25. What is the new distance?

2. The distance was 40″ SID and the mR was 7. The mR was changed to 1.75. What distance must be used?

3. A distance of 40″ SID and 20 mAs was used for a specific technique. If the distance is changed to 72″ SID, what MAS is needed?

4. What is the square root of 5184?

5. If an mA of 500 is used with a time of .05 second, what is the MA if the time is changed to .5 second? Consider only the mA . . . mAs will be covered separately.

6. An exposure time of 0.1 at 55″ SID was used. The distance was changed to 36″ SID. What is the new time?

7. For a technique of a specific examination, 10 mR at 48″ SID was used. The distance is to be changed to 72″ SID. What is the new mR?

8. What is the formula for the Inverse Square Law?

9. Student "A" took six abdomen radiographs, and student "B" took nine abdomen radiographs. With this information, answer the following questions.

   A. How many more radiographs did student "B" take than student "A"?

   B. Student "B" took _____times more radiographs than Student "A."

   C. Student "B" took _____of all the radiographs.

10. When a number is written like this: 36^2, what does it mean? What is the solution?

11. 72^2 equals _____ .

12. 200 mA was used at a distance of 36″ SID. The exposure time was kept constant, but the distance was changed to 72″ SID. What MA is needed to maintain density (degree of blackness) on the film?

13. Change from a 6:1 grid to a 12:1 grid. The conversion factor for 6:1 is 3, and the conversion factor for 12:1 is 5. How many times must the exposure factors be increased to make the compensation for the change in grids?

14. The number in the top position in a ratio for a fraction is called the

(a) _____ , and the number in the bottom position is called

the (b) _____.

15. For a specific technique, 20 mR was used at 40″ SID. The mR was changed to 5. What is the required distance for this change in mR?

16. What is the square root of the following numbers: (a) 2401?

_____ (b) 72? _____

See pages 143-144 in answer key to check your answers.

The 15% Rule and the Reciprocity Law

Objectives

■ ■ ■ ■ ■ ■ ■ ■ ■ ■ ■

After this unit you should be able to:

1. Convert a fraction to a decimal and a decimal to a fraction.

2. Change a decimal to a percentage and a percentage to a decimal.

3. Apply the 15% Rule to increase or decrease kilovoltage levels.

4. Make corresponding technique adjustment in mAs.

5. Discuss how the 15% Rule impacts on the resulting diagnostic image.

6. Discuss how and why the Reciprocity Law works in making radiographic technique adjustments.

7. Identify, in a radiographic technique, where the Reciprocity Law can be applied and effectively used.

FIFTEEN-PERCENT RULE

An important technical rule frequently used in radiology is called **the 15% Rule.** It is used because, first, it works, and second, the results are predictable. This level of dependability is an important consideration whenever a technique must be changed. Our professional evaluations are dependent on our ability to predict, within reasonable limits, how and in which way a technique change should be made.

Although it is important to point out that other levels of technical changes can be and are used, the 15% Rule is more frequently used and cited in the literature. If you want more information regarding the other possible technical changes that involve increasing or decreasing kilovoltage on the basis of a percent of change, refer to the bibliography.

The 15-Percent Rule has a **minimum** of three aspects that must be considered when it is put to use. These aspects are as follows:

1. Knowledge of percentages and decimals.

2. How kVp is changed.

3. How and why mAs is changed or may need to be changed when the 15% Rule is used.

The rule states that an **increase of 15% in kVp** *approximately doubles the effects* of the exposure **(mA), thus giving the film more density or blackness.**

This means that when the kVp has been increased by 15%, the mAs must be reduced to one-half its original amount.

Conversely, this rule implies that with a decrease in kVp by 15%, the mAs must be doubled if one is to maintain the original density, or blackness, level on the film.

Be aware that implied in the discussion of this rule is a basic tenant of radiographic exposure: **The kilovoltage used in the technique must adequately penetrate the subject so the film exhibits accepted levels of contrast and density.**

This basic rule is further supported by the fact that **no amount of mAs will compensate for lack of kVp.** (Burns, 1992; Bushong, 1993; Carlton-Adler, 1992; Eastman, 1979; Selman, 1985; Thompson, 1979).

Your professional judgment, in conjunction with the requirements of the radiologist in the evaluation of technique changes seen on resulting radiographs, is important in the determination of the film's diagnostic quality. Often you will have the singular responsibility of deciding the technical quality of a film; thus it is important to learn how this rule fits into the scheme of an integrated system of radiographic exposure mathematics.

Application

There is nothing mysterious about this rule. It has proven useful in technical adjustments, and the calculations are easy to learn and execute in daily practice. To apply the rule, you must know the relationship between percentages and decimals.

Recall that a percent is a part or fraction of the base number 100. The symbol for this fraction is "%."

Example: 15% is an abbreviated form of $\frac{15}{100}$.

Obviously, the symbol is easier to use.

When working with a percent, the percent must be converted to a decimal. The simplest method for this conversion is done by placing a decimal point two (2) places to the left of the decimal point in the series of numbers.

For example: Evaluate the decimal placements.

PERCENT	DECIMAL
1000	10.00
100	1.00
10	0.10
075	0.75
07500	75.00
25	0.25
15	0.15

These examples should give you a good review of decimal placement, but we can also check it out mathematically. This is how it is done:

Example: To change $\dfrac{15}{100}$ to a decimal, we must divide 15 (the numerator) by 100 (the denominator).

$$\begin{array}{r} .15 \\ 100\overline{)15.00} \\ 10\ 0 \\ \hline 50\ 0 \\ 50\ 0 \end{array}$$

(NOTE: A decimal and zeros must be added to 15 because it is smaller than the divisor.)

Answer: .15

Example: To change a decimal to a percent, drop the decimal point, move the decimal point two places to the right, and do one of two things:

Procedure: Place 15 over 100 as shown: $\dfrac{15}{100}$

or add ONLY the symbol: 15%

The symbol is more efficient.

FRACTIONS INTO DECIMALS

Fractions have been mentioned with some frequency in this book, but in this unit, the fraction is going to be dissected and evaluated. In some areas, specifically timers on most radiographic units, the lowly fraction has been replaced by the more classy and easier to use decimal.

There are many classifications of fractions, but we will concern ourselves with those fractions that are less than one. If you want more experience with fractions, there are many useful basic mathematics books, in paperback, available through the library or in bookstores.

We can multiply, add, subtract, and divide fractions, but it is much easier to perform these mathematical functions if we use decimals instead.

Example: Suppose you want to add the following fractions: 1/2; 3/4, and 1/5. If you haven't added this many fractions in a long time, you may have forgotten how to get the solution.

The easiest thing to do is convert the fractions into decimals, and you do this by division.

PROBLEM 1: What is the decimal and the percentage of the fraction 1/2?

Procedure:

Step 1: Divide the numerator by the denominator.

Step 2:

$$
\begin{array}{r}
0.5 \\
2\overline{)1.000} \\
\underline{0} \\
1\ 0
\end{array}
$$

Answer: 0.5, or 50%

PROBLEM 2: Convert 3/4 to a decimal and to a percent.

Procedure:

Step 1: Divide numerator 3 by denominator 4.

Step 2:

$$
\begin{array}{r}
0.75 \\
4\overline{)3.00} \\
3\ 0 \\
\underline{2\ 8} \\
20 \\
20
\end{array}
$$

Answer: .75, or 75%

PROBLEM 3: Change 1/5 to a decimal and a percent.

Procedure:

Step 1: Divide numerator 1 by denominator 5.

Step 2:

$$
\begin{array}{r}
0.2 \\
5\overline{)1.000} \\
\underline{0} \\
1\,0 \\
\underline{1\,0}
\end{array}
$$

Answer: 0.2, or 20%

The next step in the efficient process of using the 15% rule is to apply it to a problem involving a technical conversion.

■ *Practice Problems*

Problem 1: Increase 62 kVp at 10 mAs by 15%.

PROCEDURE:

Step 1: Multiply 62 kVp by 15%. (Remember: Convert the percent to a decimal and watch decimal places.)

$$
\begin{array}{r}
62 \\
\times .15 \\
\hline
310 \\
62 \\
\hline
930 \ (9.30) \quad \text{ANSWER:} \quad 9.3
\end{array}
$$

Step 2: Add 9.3 to original 62 kVp.

$$
\begin{array}{r}
62.0 \\
9.3 \\
\hline
71.3 \ \text{or 71 kVp is to be used.}
\end{array}
$$

Step 3: Recall that an increase of 15% in kVp means the mAs must be halved. Thus if 10 mAs was originally used, it now becomes 5 mAs.

ANSWER:

   71 (or 70) kVp at 5 mAs

Problem 2: Your technique is 75 kVp at 25 mAs. Decrease the kVp by 15%.

PROCEDURE:

Step 1:

$$
\begin{array}{r}
75 \\
\times \ .15 \\
\hline
375 \\
75 \\
\hline
11.25
\end{array}
$$

Step 2:

$$
\begin{array}{r}
75.00 \\
-11.25 \\
\hline
63.75 \ \text{or 64 kVp}
\end{array}
$$

The new mAs must be doubled to compensate for decrease in kVp.

ANSWER:

64 kVp at 50 mAs.

In daily practice you may be asked to evaluate a radiographic technique that you have not directly worked with.

EVALUATE THE ABOVE PROBLEM, AND ANSWER THIS QUESTION.

Is this correct? Yes _____   No _____

Some machines may not allow incremental changes of less than 1 kVp; thus the fractional amounts are rounded off to the nearest whole number. (Carlton-Adler, 1992; Thompson, 1979)

Problem 3: Your technique is 52 kVp and 100 mAs; you want to increase the kVp by 15%.

PROCEDURE:

Step 1: Multiply 52 kVp by 15% (Remember to convert percent to a decimal.)

$$\begin{array}{r} 52 \\ \times .15 \\ \hline 260 \\ 52 \\ \hline \end{array}$$

ANSWER:

7.80, thus, the original 52 kVp will increase by 7.8 or 8 kVp

Step 2: Add: 52 + 8 = 60 kVp

Step 3: With this increase in kVp, you will need to adjust the mAs by 1/2 (or 50%).

ANSWER:

50 mAs at 60 kVp.

THE RECIPROCITY LAW

The Reciprocity Law is a complex and useful law in the physics of radiology, but the mathematical applications are straight-forward and relatively easy to learn and use. The discussion in this book will be limited to and focused on the mathematical applications as related to mAs (milliamps-seconds). For more complex descriptions and discussions, refer to the references listed at the end of this section.

The **Reciprocity Law** states that, within reasonable limits, the optical density or blackness on the film can be maintained as long as the mAs is constant.

Mathematically, the Reciprocity Law can be expressed in the terms milliamps-seconds (mAs). The relationship looks like this:

$$\text{Original MAS} = \text{NEW mAs}$$

In technique calculations the Reciprocity Law has a direct impact on the milliamps-seconds factors. Application of this law in equation form shows us that the products of two separate calculations can be matched even though the parameters (mA and seconds) in each factor set are different.

Examples of the Reciprocity Law as applied to mAs in Radiographic Techniques:

Technique 1: 500 mA @ .015 sec = 7.5 mAs.

Technique 2: 300 mA @ .025 sec = 7.5 mAs.

Technique 3: 250 mA @ .03 sec = 7.5 mAs.

The adjustment of mA and seconds to obtain a shorter or longer exposure time, while keeping the same mAs constant *without* an appreciable change in the visible density on the finished film, is important and useful in making quality technical factor changes.

However, a few cautionary notes are necessary regarding the most broad use and interpretation of this law.

Both student and practicing radiographers should be familiar with the limitations of the Reciprocity Law that are governed by the following parameters:

1. Effective kVp range.

2. Exposure time limitations.

3. Film-screen combination speed limitations and film sensitivity levels.

4. Effective mA range.

5. Tube-rating levels.

These factors, especially at the extreme ends of the available ranges, may result in a failure of the Reciprocity Law. Failure of this reciprocal relationship happens between the intensity of the exposure and the duration of the exposure and can occur even though the mAs product is the same. (Examples: very long or very short exposure times, and when intensifying screens are used.)

This law contributes greatly to the radiographer's ability to manipulate techniques and get consistent results, especially with respect to milliamps-seconds (mAs) adjustments.

The major requirement for this relationship to work consistently is use of x-ray equipment that has been competently designed and properly calibrated. (Burns, 1992; Carlton-Adler, 1992; Hiss, 1993; Selman, 1982; Thompson, 1979).

RESEARCH PROJECTS

You may choose either one of these projects, or you may combine aspects of both subjects. See the specific instructions.

Project 1: Fifteen-Percent Rule

The 15% Rule will serve you well in daily decision-making when technical factors need some adjustments, but to more fully understand how it functions, evaluate each of the preceding practice problems against other aspects of percentage of kVp and mAs increase or decrease. List the advantages and disadvantages and summarize your interpretations into a two- or three-page paper.

Study Questions

Use these questions to guide you in your research and in writing your paper.

1. Is the 15% Rule a standard for all kVp settings?

2. What are the limitations, if any, on the use of this rule?

3. Could you use the 15% Rule as a primary control over density or blackness of the film? Why or why not?

Project 2: The Reciprocity Law

You are encouraged to learn all you can about the Reciprocity Law, because understanding how it works is integral to helping make interpretation and evaluation of technical judgments easier. List the advantages and disadvantages encountered in this law. The study questions will guide you in your research and as you write your paper.

Study Questions

1. Why would the Reciprocity Law fail?

2. Why is the Reciprocity Law less apt to fail in a direct exposure technique?

3. What areas of the technique range would be the most susceptible to failure of the Reciprocity Law?

4. Why would the use of intensifying screens in a radiographic procedure be susceptible to failure of the Reciprocity Law?

(Useful References: Burns, 1992; Bushong, 1993; Carlton-Adler, 1992; Meredith-Massey, 1977; Selman, 1985; Thompson, 1979).

U N I T 8

Integrated Radiographic Exposure Practice Problems and Research Projects

Objectives
■ ■ ■ ■ ■ ■ ■ ■ ■ ■ ■

After completion of this unit, you should be able to:

1. Evaluate the mathematical changes necessary to complete the technique change or changes.

2. Do the necessary calculations to make the necessary technique change or changes.

3. Discuss the reasons for selecting a technical change or series of changes.

4. Use the library to find reference sources and compile your research notes and bibliography.

5. Write a research paper, minimum two to three pages, about kVp, Source-Image-Distances, motion unsharpness, 15% Rule, or the Reciprocity Law.

This unit is designed to help you effectively evaluate, analyze, and integrate the information and procedures necessary in working with radiographic exposure technique change problems.

The task of evaluating radiographic technique problems has been made easier by using a system of dissecting each problem and guiding you through steps necessary to solve the problem. This system will give you an opportunity to apply what you have learned thus far, integrate the information, and think analytically.

The emphasis on changing one factor at a time remains true as each problem step is evaluated; however, when you have completed the necessary steps in a technique change, you may find that more than one factor has been affected by the initial change. This is a key point in mathematics of radiographic system; it is an integrated system.

■ *Practice Problems*

■

Problem 1: Evaluate technique #1 for changes, incorporate changes for technique #2 with an increase in the kVp by 15%, and make the corresponding changes in the new technique.

SHOW ALL CALCULATIONS/FORMULAS

TECHNIQUE 1	TECHNIQUE 2
65 kVp	_____ kVp
100 mA	_____ mA
.1 sec	_____ sec
10 mAs	_____ mAs
40" SID	_40"_ SID
Screen Speed 100	Screen Speed 100
8:1 Grid	8:1 Grid

PROCEDURE:

Step 1: Extract vital information and use 15% Rule.

Original kVp $65 \times .15 = 9.75$

Add original kVp 65 and 9.75

ANSWER:

New kVp = 74.7 or 75 kVp

Step 2: Think about any other changes that must be made to keep the density on the new film comparable to the density on the original.

The **15% rule** states: **"With an increase in kVp by 15%, the mAs must be decreased by 50% or by 1/2."**

Likewise, with a 15% decrease in kVp, the mAs should be increased two times. Generally, this rule will work UNLESS the kVp is insufficient to effectively penetrate the object. (Burns, 1992; Bushong, 1992; Carlton-Adler, 1992; Hiss, 1993; Selman, 1985; Thompson, 1979).

Step 3: Choose one answer from the following list for Technique #1 changes that will be best suited to stop motion, maintain the density, and provide high-quality recorded detail, that is, geometrical and visual sharpness of the image:

(1) 100 mA at 0.05 (1/20) sec = 5 mAs

(2) 200 mA at 0.025 (1/40) sec = 5 mAs

(3) 50 mA at 0.1 (1/10) sec = 5 mAs

(4) 20 mA at 0.25 (1/4) sec = 5 mAs

ANSWER:

200 mA at .025 (1/40) sec

Why select this answer? Though each of the techniques available will compensate for the 15% increase in kVp, the radiographer must consider other factors in selecting the technique.

These factors are:

• Large vs small focal spot

• Exposure time

• Tube ratings

• Radiation exposure

• Motion unsharpness

• Screen speed

• Film speed

If involuntary motion is a problem, the best technique would be one with the shortest exposure time even if a larger focal spot must be used. Why be concerned with the size of the focal spot?

As you recall, the smaller focal spot will give you greater geometric sharpness. Can you explain this statement?

Additionally, the higher kVp used in the technique change will result in less blooming or broadening of the focal spot, providing tube limits are not exceeded. Blooming, or an increase in the size of the focal spot, occurs when the tube current (mA) is increased. (Burns, 1992; Cullinan-Cullinan, 1994; Hiss, 1993; Selman, 1985; Thompson, 1979).

You should consider technique selections that fit into the safe ranges of both tube ratings and lowered radiation exposure to the patient, bearing in mind that these factors are separate calculations based on other specifications.

The best advice: Keep your techniques within the safe limits of the tube ratings.

Manufacturers provide tube rating charts with x-ray tubes that allow the radiographer to evaluate the technique against the heating and cooling capacity times of the materials used in the construction of the x-ray tube.

Assessment of the tube rating is a multiplication problem that comes under the heading of **Heat Units.**

Each x-ray tube anode has the ability to carry a limited amount of heat. If the heat limit capacity is exceeded, the anode will be damaged.

Heat Units are defined in a basic equation:

Single Phase:

$$\text{Heat Units (H.U.)} = KV \times MA \times Sec$$

Three Phase/Six Pulse:

$$\text{H.U.} \times 1.35 = \text{Heat Units}$$

Three Phase/12-Pulse:

$$\text{H.U.} \times 1.41 = \text{Heat Units}$$

This equation represents energy that must be evaluated in relation to the type of generator used, size of the focal spot and target, as well as the length of time it takes for the anode to cool.

Extended discussion on the application of the formula for Heat Units will not be handled in this book except to introduce you to the basic formula and compensation factors.

Be aware that manufacturers of x-ray machines provide these useful charts. The radiographer's job is to be able to calculate HEAT UNITS and evaluate the technique against the information on the tube rating charts.

Some useful references are Bushong, 1993; Carlton-Adler, 1992; Cullinan-Cullinan, 1994; Hiss, 1993; Meredith-Massey, 1979; Selman, 1985.

Radiation exposure is also a consideration. The primary goals of a competent radiographer should be to use all precautions to reduce radiation exposure. While there are many ways to ensure optimum radiation safety, some of these precautions are:

- Proper and consistent use of gonadal shielding.
- Accurate collimation or beam restriction of radiation field.
- Functional technique charts to eliminate repeat examinations.
- Calibrated machines.
- Daily quality control on automatic film processors.
- Proper filtration.

This list is not intended to be a complete list of the various aspects concerning radiation exposure considerations. Check the bibliography for more sources of information on this important topic.

In Problem 2, the significant technique change involves evaluating the change of speed of the intensifying screens; thus before you proceed, read through this basic information about Relative Speed of intensifying screens.

The changes in this technique require changing any factors that may be affected by use of a faster or slower speed intensifying screen. A chart that will give you some basic information is provided in this unit, but you should check screen and film manufacturer information for the most accurate conversion factors.

The Relative Speed of Screens is an **arbitrary number** that must be considered within the context of the system used in your department, although this chart will give you enough information so you can learn to make the basic technical conversions.

In daily practice, you must know the Basic Relative Speed of your imaging system, which includes types of intensifying screens, film, and processing speeds.

Relative Screen Speed numbers

1200	150
800	125
600	100
400	80
300	60
250	50

Speeds listed in descending order. The numbers on this chart have been extracted from the following sources and do not indicate all possible combinations of film and screens. (Burns, 1992; Bushong, 1992; Carlton-Adler, 1992; Cullinan-Cullinan, 1994; Technical information sheets: E.I. DuPont and Eastman Kodak, 1993; Selman, 1985).

Problem 2:

TECHNIQUE 3	adjust to	TECHNIQUE 4
70 kVp		70 kVp
100 mA		100 mA
.1 (1/10) sec		_____ sec
10 mAs		_____ mAs
40″ SID		40″ SID
Screen Speed 50		Screen Speed 100

The original mAs in Technique 4 is 10. First, notice that the speed of intensifying screens has changed. What is the new MAS for the faster screen system?

PROCEDURE:

Step 1: Write the formula for the increased speed in intensifying screens, and extract the vital information.

$$MAS_2 = \frac{\text{Relative Screen Speed}_1 \times mAs_1}{\text{Relative Screen Speed}_2}$$

$$MAS_2 = \frac{50 \times 10}{100} = \frac{500}{100} = 5$$

ANSWER:

5 MAS

We can take a closer look at our technique once the change in mAs has been made to make sure we have kept the proper inverse proportional relationship.

Step 2: The relationship of mAs and screen speed is an inverse proportion. Recall "the product of the **extremes** equals the product of the **means**." Write the formula for checking accuracy of a proportion.

$$mAs_1 : MAS_2 : : \text{Screen Speed}_2 : \text{Screen Speed}_1$$

| 10 | 5 | 100 | 50 |

Multiply the Extremes: Result: _____

Multiply the Means: Result: _____

Answer for Extremes and Means: 500. Because the extremes and the means are equal, assume your new MAS is accurate.

Step 3: What new exposure time is needed in your technique to equal 5 mAs?

Step 4: Write the formula to calculate exposure time in seconds (with constant MA).

$$\frac{mAs_1}{MAS_2} = \frac{T_2}{t_1}$$

Step 5: Extract the vital information and put numbers into the formula.

$$\frac{5}{10} = \frac{X}{.1}$$

Step 6: Cancel where appropriate.

$$.1 \times \frac{5}{10} = \frac{X}{\cancel{X}} \times \cancel{X}$$

Step 7: Complete calculations.

$$X = .1 \times \frac{5}{10} = \frac{.5}{10} = .05 \text{ sec}$$

ANSWER:

.05 Sec at 100 mA.

Step 8: Determine new milliamps-seconds:

Step 9: Write formula and extract vital information.

$$mAs = mA \times sec \text{ (exposure time)}$$

$$mAs = 100 \times .05$$

ANSWER:

5 mAs

Problem 3:

TECHNIQUE 5	adjust to	TECHNIQUE 6
70 kVp		70 kVp
100 mA		100 mA
.1 sec		_____ sec
10 mAs		_____ mAs
40″ SID		36″ SID
Screen speed 50		Screen speed 50
8:1 focused grid		8:1 focused grid

The original technique was satisfactory, but the patient was moved to a radiographic unit with a shorter, but fixed, SID. Make the corrections in the exposure factors.

PROCEDURE:

Step 1: List technique changes. Write formulas and extract vital information for each of these changes.

- Distance
- mAs
- Time

Step 2: Because the distance is changed, the mAs must be adjusted. The formula is:

$$\frac{mAs_1}{SID_1^2} = \frac{MAS_2}{SID_2^2}$$

OR

$$\frac{mAs_1}{MAS_2} = \frac{SID_1^2}{SID_2^2}$$

Choose the rule that governs this problem.

    A. mAs and distance are inversely proportional.

    B. mAs and distance cannot be calculated in a ratio.

    C. mAs and distance are directly proportional.

ANSWER:

        mAs and distance are directly proportional.

Step 3: Extract the vital information and write the formula

$$mAs_1 = 10$$

$$MAS_2 = X$$

$$SID_1^2 = 40^2$$

$$SID_2^2 = 36^2$$

Formula to be used: Note how this formula is set up. What is different about it? Why will it work?

$$\frac{mAs_1}{SID_1^2} = \frac{MAS_2}{SID_2^2}$$

Step 4:

$$\frac{10}{40^2} = \frac{X}{36^2}$$

Step 5: Liberate the "X" in the equation.

$$36^2 \cdot \frac{10}{40^2} = \frac{X}{\cancel{36^2}} \cdot \cancel{36^2}$$

Step 6: The problem now looks like this:

$$X = \frac{(36 \times 36) \times 10}{(40 \times 40)} = \frac{12960}{1600} = 8.1$$

ANSWER:

    8.1 mAs.

The Shortcut Method involves cancelling and reducing to the lowest numbers. This makes doing the calculations very easy.

$$X = \frac{\overset{(9 \times 9)}{(\cancel{36} \times \cancel{36})} \times 10}{\underset{(10 \times 10)}{(\cancel{40} \times \cancel{40})}} = \frac{810}{100}$$

Cancel the extra zeros.

$$X = 81.0 \text{ divided by } 10 = 8.1$$

ANSWER:

8.1 mAs

If you cannot obtain 8 mAs on your machine, use 10 mAs instead. The addition of 2 mAs will hardly be discernible unless you are working with kVp levels lower than 45.

You can double-check your calculations by using the process: "The product of the means should be equal to the product of the extremes."

$$\text{extremes : MEANS : : MEANS : extremes}$$

$$mAs_1 : \quad SID_1^2 \quad : : \quad MAS_2 \quad : SID_2^2$$

$$10 : \quad 40_1^2 \quad : : \quad 8.1 \quad : 36_2^2$$

If you "rounded off" 8.1 mAs to 8 mAs, and multiplied (40×40), the result is 12,800. On occasion, you may encounter answers with slight differences due to "round-off errors," but this is of little concern. This method, while it works as a double-check on your calculations, is also a way to do the problems.

Step 7: mA and Time selections

With the mAs change made because of distance adjustments, you will need to select the best combination of mA and seconds (exposure time).

The selection of a new mAs is done by the following method:

$$\textbf{Formula: Seconds} = \frac{\textbf{mAs}}{\textbf{mA}}$$

Step 8: Extract the vital information and place in the formula

$$X = \frac{8}{100}$$

Step 9: Divide or reduce to the lowest terms.

$$4 \mid \frac{8}{100} = \frac{2}{25} \text{ or}$$

Your division will look like the following:

$$100\overline{)8.00} \quad .08 \text{ seconds}$$

ANSWER:

Final technique looks like this:

70 kVp	36" SID
100 mA	Screen Speed 100
.08 sec	8 mAs
8:1 Focused Grid	

Problem 4: Evaluate Technique 7 and make changes for Technique 8.

TECHNIQUE 7   adjusted to   TECHNIQUE 8

TECHNIQUE 7	TECHNIQUE 8
60 kVp	_____ kVp
300 mA	300 mA
0.03 sec	0.016 sec
10 mAs	_____ mAs
40" SID	40" SID
Table Top	Table Top
Screen Speed 50	Screen Speed 50

You have changed the exposure time in Technique 8. Make the necessary calculations and adjustments.

PROCEDURE:

Remember the following:

1. Write formulas and extract vital information.

2. Show the calculations.

Technique factor changes include:

• mAs

• kVp

What is the primary rule that governs mAs and kVp relationships?

A. 30% rule for kVp levels over 75.

B. Do not change the technique.

C. Use screen speed 1200.

D. 15% Rule.

ANSWER:

For this problem, the 15% Rule has been applied. Other percentage changes in kVp can be used, depending on the kVp level. Check references for additional information about kVp changes.

Step 1: Calculate the mAs.

Step 2: Write the formula and set up the problem.

$$mAs = MA \times Seconds \text{ (Exposure Time)}$$

$$X = 300 \times 0.016 = 4.8 \text{ or } 5 \text{ mAs}$$

Step 5: Calculate the new kVp using the 15% Rule.

$$\text{Original kVp} \times 15\% = \textbf{new kVp factor}$$

- To *increase* kVp: Original kVp + new kVp factor

- To *decrease* kVp: Original kVp − new kVp factor

Recall that a 50% reduction in mAs will require at least a 15% increase in kVp, although slight variations may be necessary depending on kVp range. Additionally, a change in kVp is likely to change the contrast levels, although this change may be advantageous.

Some useful references that have expanded discussion on other aspects of the 15% Rule are Burns, 1992; Bushong, 1993; Carroll, 1993; Carlton-Adler, 1992; Cullinan-Cullinan, 1994; Selman, 1985; Thompson, 1979.

kVP ADJUSTMENTS

Original kVp = 60   New kVp = ____?____

Original mAs = 10   New mAs = 5

With a decrease in mAs by 50%, you can use the 15% Rule, which means an increase in kVp is needed to compensate for the decreased mAs.

Recall: Original kVp × .15% = kVp factor 60 kVp times .15 = 9.00, the kVp factor.

Original kVp + kVp factor = New kVp.

        60   + 9.00   = 69 kVp.

ANSWER:

Your adjusted technique now looks like this:

69 kVp	40″ SID
300 mA	Screen Speed 50
0.016	Table Top Exposure
5 mAs	No Grid

Problem 5: The new technique results from a change in the mAs

TECHNIQUE 9	adjusted to	TECHNIQUE 10
70 kVp		70 kVp
200 mA		200 mA
0.2 sec		_____ sec
40 mAs		160 mAs
36″ SID		_____ SID
12:1 Focused grid		12:1 Focused Grid
Screen Speed 100		Screen Speed 100

There are three major changes in this technique, but remember to change one factor at a time.

PROCEDURE:

Again, do the following:

1. List technique changes.

2. Write formulas and extract vital information.

3. Show calculations.

Technique changes include:

- Exposure Time (seconds)

- mAs

- SID

Step 1: Formula for calculation of the new exposure time.

$$(\text{Exposure Time}) \text{ Seconds} = \frac{\text{mAs}}{\text{MA}}$$

Step 2: Extract the vital information to adjust exposure time.

$$\text{Exposure Time} = X \text{ (seconds)}$$

$$\text{mAs} = 160$$

$$\text{MA} = 200$$

Step 3: Set up problem.

$$\text{Seconds} = \frac{\text{mAs}}{\text{MA}}$$

$$X = \frac{160}{200} = .8 \text{ sec}$$

or as an option, you may compute the problem to get the fraction equivalent of the decimal.

Example:

$$4 \,\Big|\, \frac{160}{200} = \frac{4}{5} \text{ sec}$$

Step 4: To calculate the mAs, write the formula, then insert the numbers and calculate.

$$\text{mAs} = \text{MA} \times \text{seconds (exposure time)}$$

$$X = 200 \times .8 = 160 \text{ mAs}$$

or you may wish to calculate the problem using this method.

$$X = 200 \times \frac{4}{5} = \frac{800}{5} = 160 \text{ mAs}$$

ANSWER:

Your emerging technique becomes:

70 kVp	36" SID
200 mA	12:1 Focused Grid
0.8 second	Screen Speed 100
160 mAs	

The 160 mAs setting, 0.8 second at 200 mA, may not be fast enough to stop involuntary motion.

Exposure time and motion, both voluntary and involuntary, are in continual conflict; thus the radiographer must select x-ray exposure time values that will eliminate motion unsharpness on the film. As we look at this technique change, check the exposure time and the mA.

Think about the techniques that are presented. Do you think 0.8 second at 200 mA (160 mAs) is sufficiently fast enough to stop unsharpness caused by involuntary motion? What can you do with technique changes to stop motion unsharpness?

Recall that the Reciprocity Law and the 15% Rule make it possible for the radiographer to manipulate technical factors that will result in the best possible recorded images. You might increase the mA to 600, for instance, which will mean the exposure time must be adjusted to accommodate the mA change. For practice, do the calculations for the new exposure time with the new mA.

The adjustment of mA and exposure time are accomplished with the use of the following formula and calculations. Study the formula and work through the problem as it has been set up. This practice will help you learn to make these technique adjustments more easily.

$$\text{SECONDS} = \frac{\text{mAs}}{\text{MA}}$$

$$\text{SECONDS} = \frac{160}{600} = .267 \text{ or } .27 \text{ sec}$$

Your mAs value becomes: **mAs = mA × seconds**

$$X = 600 \times .267 = 160.2 \text{ or } 160 \text{ mAs}$$

There are other portions of this problem yet to be solved, but before we get into those solutions, we need to pause and do a little in-depth study and review of the technical changes we have used thus far.

The new distance is unknown but will be set according to the new mAs values.

PROCEDURE:

Recall that in calculating distances, we are working with a squared number; thus we will need to find the square root.

Step 1: Write the formula for mAs-Distance:

$$\frac{\text{mAs}_1}{\text{SID}_1^2} = \frac{\text{MAS}_2}{\text{SID}_2^2}$$

Step 2: Extract the vital information.

$$\text{mAs}_1 = 40$$

$$\text{MAS}_2 = 160$$

$$\text{SID}_1^2 = 36^2$$

$$\text{SID}_2^2 = X^2$$

Step 3: Set up the problem with the correct numbers needed for the problem:

$$X = \frac{40}{36^2} = \frac{160}{X^2}$$

Step 4: Invert sides of the equation so the "X" will be in the numerator position for easy calculation.

$$\frac{36^2}{40} = \frac{X^2}{160}$$

Step 5: Liberate the "X."

$$160 \times \frac{(36 \times 36)}{40} = \frac{X^2}{\cancel{160}} \times \cancel{160}$$

Step 6: Cancel where appropriate. Your equation should now look like this:

$$X^2 = \frac{160(36 \times 36)}{40} = \frac{207360}{40}$$

$$X^2 = 207360 \div 40$$

$$X^2 = 5184$$

Because X^2 is a squared number, you must find the square root of 5184. Use a calculator to find the answer.

ANSWER:

X = 72" SID

This last practice problem should be considered when you are doing the research and as you write the associated paper. Study questions and some useful references are given to help you.

RESEARCH PROJECT 1: MILLIAMPERAGE-KILOVOLTAGE ADJUSTMENT USING THE 15% RULE

While the exposure time can be reduced by increasing the mA, you might try manipulating the technique by adjusting the kVp through the 15% Rule. Because this rule is useful, and assuming the original technique is satisfactory, it is important to know how using this rule may affect the levels of contrast and density on the film. But before leaping into the use of this rule, a research project is in order.

To help you with your research, here are some useful references. (Burns, 1992; Bushong, 1993; Carlton-Adler, 1992; Carroll, 1993; Cullinan-Cullinan, 1994; Hiss, 1993; Selman, 1985; Thompson, 1979).

Prepare a research paper about the technique adjustment processes that involve changing kVp through use of the 15% Rule. Investigate and evaluate the theories and physics of the changes that occur when kVp levels are increased versus decreased.

Use the following study questions as a guide in the development of your paper. You are to assume that you are the teacher; thus the person who reads what you've written is your student. Write your paper for this student. Be thorough but concise, and adhere to the basic principles for writing a scientific paper.

Questions to Consider:

1. Briefly discuss both increase and decrease in kVp levels in conjunction with the use of the 15% rule.

2. The contrast and density levels on the recorded image will change when you change kVp and mAs. Discuss some of the expected changes that are visible to the unaided eye of the radiographer.

3. Briefly explain how mAs primarily affects the visible levels of density and/or contrast on the recorded image.

4. What happens at the x-ray target? What is different or similar about the x-rays that are formed?

5. Explain the attenuation of x-rays when they pass through various types of tissues found in the body, such as bones, hair, fingernails, intestines, fat, muscle, air-filled, and so forth. Explain how the recorded images differ in appearance (not size or shape), and why these differences occur.

6. Briefly describe or illustrate the interaction of the x-rays as they interact with the intensifying screens.

7. How does the x-ray/intensifying screen interaction affect the film?

8. Explain the relevance of the Reciprocity Law in technical changes.

Your paper should contain a well-stated hypothesis, literature review, materials and methods, discussion, conclusion, and bibliography.

Your discussion and conclusion should reflect your opinion based on the facts you've collected and/or observed through the literature research readings, clinical experiences, or laboratory exercises.

Once you have completed this research paper, you will be well-prepared to solve the following problems; however, our first problem will be the conclusion of Problem 5, which was begun before the research project was introduced.

■ *Practice Problems—continued*

■ *Problem 5: Conclusion*

As we continue to solve Problem 5, we can use the 15% Rule to increase the kVp, which will allow us to decrease the MAS.

To recap the procedure, the increase of kVp by 15% works like this:

- .15 times 70 = 10.5 (kVp factor)

    Original kVp (70) + kVp factor (10.5)

- 10.5 + 70 kVp = 80.5 or 81 kVp.

With this change in kVp, the 15% Rule states that you must compensate for the increase in kVp by lowering the mAs by two times, or 50%.

Milliamps-Seconds Adjustment: Once the kVp has been correctly changed, adjust the mAs by 50%, or 1/2, as dictated by the rule.

The problem will be calculated with both a decimal and a fraction so you can see how each operates within the system.

mAs calculations with a fraction: 160 mAs divided by 2 = 80 mAs

or the **preferred** method: mAs calculations with a decimal:

Answer:

160 mAs times .50 = 80 adjusted mAs.

Now that you have adjusted **BOTH** the kVp and the mAs, you will need to recalculate your exposure time value.

The method we use will keep the mA at 600 and adjust the exposure time to match the reduced mAs. As you may recall, the original mA was 200, but an increase to 600 mA seemed like an excellent way to reduce the length of the exposure time. (Note: This sentence has a subtle reference to the Reciprocity Law.)

Formula: mAs = mA × Seconds:

Seconds = mAs divided by mA

$$X = \frac{80}{600}$$

Answer:

0.13 seconds exposure time

If you recalculate your mAs with the new exposure time value, that is, mAs = mA × seconds, your answer will be 79.9, or 80 after rounding off the number.

The faster exposure time will help stop involuntary motion.

(Useful References: Burns, 1992; Bushong, 1993; Carlton-Adler, 1992; Cullinan-Cullinan, 1994; Carroll, 1993; Hiss, 1993; Meredith-Massey, 1977; Selman, 1985; Thompson, 1979).

ANSWER:

Your FINAL technique becomes:

81 kVp	72″ SID
600 mA	12:1 Focused Grid
.13 sec	Screen Speed 100
80 mAs	

With respect to the change in Source-Image-Distance as a method to compensate for other technique changes, it is doubtful that such a method would be used. However, this problem illustrates that a change in **DISTANCE** can be used to compensate for other technique changes and still retain the diagnostic integrity of the film.

This problem also illustrates that when a distance is changed, the intensity of the x-ray beam is changed as the distance is squared. This problem can be manipulated in several different ways, and various changes can be considered, such as change in kVp, mAs, or distance, and so forth.

(Useful references: Burns, 1992; Carlton-Adler, 1992; Carroll, 1993; Bushong, 1993; Hiss, 1993; Selman, 1985.)

RESEARCH PROJECT 2: TECHNIQUE EVALUATION

Objectives: Following the study and participation in these research problems, you should:

1. Be able to design a set of experimental radiographic exposure problems.

2. Work within your group to develop a research and discussion protocol.

3. Gather supporting documentation to support your research and findings.

4. Write a paper on the results of your findings.

5. OPTIONAL: Prepare the results of your findings to be presented to your class, and include any useful hand-out material for distribution.

Form small study groups, and develop a protocol for a panel discussion, a scientific paper, or research project to study and explain the various technical changes in a radiographic exposure problem designed by your group. The final result from your designer problem should show at least three major technical adjustments.

With a phantom or aluminum step-wedge, adjust the kVp, mAs, and SID and evaluate the differences in the appearance of the resulting films from both techniques, both visually and with a densitometer.

Discuss the findings of your research project and be able to support your findings and conclusions by your research and by citing the works of other experts in radiology.

Documentation of sources should follow standard bibliographic notations. Use parenthetical notation format within the paper. Be prepared to give your findings in an oral report based on your paper.

RESEARCH PROJECT 3: MOTION UNSHARPNESS

Note: This experiment needs the approval of your instructor.

Design and carry out a laboratory experiment that demonstrates the problems of motion unsharpness, how the problems can be solved, and how motion can be used to an advantage in various radiological procedures.

Geometric and motion unsharpness are conditions that must be carefully controlled, but in some instances, both motion and nonstandard Object-Film-Distance or Source-Object-Film Distances can be manipulated to demonstrate specific diagnostic problems. Some of these situations involve specialized techniques.

Research the various aspects of geometric and motion unsharpness and write a paper that describes the historical and current clinical or research applications.

Document your paper, and cite examples or provide examples or illustrations of the clinical applications of geometric or motion unsharpness.

You may focus on one specific area of geometric unsharpness used in diagnostic evaluations, but regardless of how you focus your paper, it should reflect your general understanding of the concepts and applications.

A word of caution: *Do not,* under any circumstances, expose a patient to get an experimental film that demonstrates involuntary motion or geometric unsharpness.

With that background, let's return to the problems.

■ *Practice Problems—continued*

Problem 6: Multiple changes in the original technique reinforce the idea of an integrated system of mathematics of exposure. Remember: Change only one factor at a time.

TECHNIQUE 11	adjusted to	TECHNIQUE 12
75 kVp		75 kVp
400 mA		_____ mA
0.05 sec		0.1 sec
20 mAs		_____ mAs
8:1 Focused Grid		5:1 Focused Grid
50″ SID		72″ SID
Screen Speed 250		Screen Speed 250

No matter how hard we try, there will always be those situations that will test your acumen in making technique changes. Look these techniques over carefully, and begin the challenge. You have the skills to successfully tackle these problems.

PROCEDURE:

Do the following:

1. List the technique changes.

2. Write the formulas and extract the vital information.

3. Show calculations.

The technique factor changes include:

• mA

• mAs

• Grid Ratio

• Distance change

Step 1: Write the formula for mA.

$$mA = \frac{mAs}{Seconds\ (Exposure\ Time)}$$

Step 2: Extract the vital information to adjust the mA

$$mA = X$$

$$mAs = 20$$

$$Seconds = 0.1\ (New\ Exposure\ Time)$$

Step 3: Set up the equation and compute:

$$mA = \frac{20}{0.1}$$

$$mA = 20 \times \frac{10}{1}$$

ANSWER:

$$mA = 200\ (mAs = 20)$$

Adjusted Technique 12 looks like this:

75 kVp	5:1 Focused Grid
200 mA	72″ SID
0.1 seconds	Screen Speed 250
20 mAs	

Step 4: Evaluate original Technique 11 and compare it with Technique 12. Proceed with making the grid ratio change. Write the formula for grid conversion.

$$Grid\ Conversion\ Factor = \frac{New\ Grid\ Factor}{Original\ Grid\ Factor}$$

$$New\ mAs = Grid\ Conversion\ Factor \times Original\ mAs$$

Step 5: Extract vital information:

$$New\ Grid\ (5:1)\ Factor = 2$$

$$Original\ Grid\ (8:1)\ Factor = 4$$

Step 6: Set up equation for changing Grid Ratios.

$$New\ mAs = \frac{2}{4} = 0.5 \times Original\ mAs$$

$$New\ mAs = 0.5 \times 20$$

ANSWER:

10 mAs

Step 7: Adjust the mA to accommodate the new mAs.

$$mA = \frac{mAs}{Time}$$

$$mA = \frac{10}{.1}$$

$$mA = 10 \times \frac{10}{1} = 100 \text{ mA}$$

Step 8: Check mAs: mAs = mA × Time

$$mAs = 100 \times .1 = 10 \text{ mAs}$$

Consider the level of mA and time. It may be more beneficial to increase the mA and decrease the exposure time even if a larger focal spot might be used. Recall you can check on the tube rating factors to see which focal spot can be safely used.

By **increasing the mA four times** and adjusting the exposure time to obtain 10 mAs, we will have the following:

Step 9: Multiply the original 100 mA by 4

ANSWER:

400 mA

Step 10: Determine the new exposure time and write the formula.

$$\text{Exposure Time} = \frac{mAs}{mA}$$
$$\text{Exposure Time} = \frac{10}{400}$$

ANSWER:

0.025 seconds

Step 11: Double check the mAs. It must match the mAs in Technique 12. Your formula for determining the new mAs is:

$$mAs = mA \times Time$$

$$mAs = 400 \times .025$$

ANSWER:

10 mAs

If you prefer to work with fractions, the mAs can also be calculated as follows:

$$mAs = 400 \times \frac{1}{40} = \frac{400}{40} = 10 \text{ mAs}$$

ANSWER:

Your emerging new technique is:

75 kVp	5:1 focused grid
400 mA	72″ SID
0.025 sec	Screen Speed 250
10 mAs	

Your final technique adjustment is distance (SID).

Step 12: Write the formula for distance and mAs.

$$\frac{mAs_1}{MAS_2} = \frac{SID_1^2}{SID_2^2}$$

Step 13: Extract the vital information.

$$mAs_1 = 10$$
$$MAS_2 = X$$
$$SID_1^2 = 50″$$
$$SID_2^2 = 72″$$

Step 14: Set up the equation.

$$\frac{10}{X} = \frac{50^2}{72^2}$$

Step 15: Invert and cancel to liberate "X" for easier calculation.

$$\cancel{10} \cdot \frac{X}{\cancel{10}} = \frac{72^2}{50^2} \cdot 10$$

Step 16: Continue the calculations.

$$X = \frac{(72 \times 72)10}{(50 \times 50)} = \frac{51840}{2500}$$

ANSWER:

20.736 which = 20 or 21 mAs.

As a result of the compensation for the increased distance required in Technique 12, the mAs has doubled from 10 to 20; thus you must **either** increase the mA **or** the time to make the exposure match the new mAs, which is your final adjustment for the SID change. (Do not change the kVp.)

Step 17: Try doubling the mA.

$$mA = 400 \times 2 = 800 \text{ mA at } 0.025 \text{ sec}$$

Now, calculate the mAs:

$$mAs = mA \times Time$$

$$mAs = 800 \times 0.025 \text{ sec}$$

ANSWER:

20 mAs

OR if you want, you can try an alternative calculations method: Leave the mA at 400 and double the exposure time.

$$Exposure\ Time = \frac{1}{40} \times 2 = \frac{2}{40}$$

Reduce to lowest terms:

$$2 \left| \frac{2}{40} = \frac{1}{20} \right.$$

In decimal form: $0.025 \times 2 = 0.05$ seconds

$$mAs = mA \times Exposure\ Time\ (Seconds)$$

$$mAs = 400 \times .05 = \frac{400}{20}$$

ANSWER:

20 mAs

The Final Adjusted technique becomes:

75 kVp	5:1 Focused Grid for 72″ SID
800 mA	72″ SID
0.025 sec	Screen Speed 250
20 mAs	

To check the calculations of the preceding problem, proceed in the following manner.

$$mAs_1 : MAS_2 :: SID_1^2 : SID_2^2$$

$$10\ :\ 20\ ::\ 50^2\ :\ 72^2$$

$$10 \times (72 \times 72) = 51840$$

$$20 \times (50 \times 50) = 50000$$

If you are concerned about the difference in the answers, check your calculations by including ALL of the numbers in the above mAs_2 calculations: $20.736 \times (50 \times 50) = 51840$. Recall that 20.736 was rounded off to be either 20 or 21. You may wish to multiply $21 \times (50 \times 50)$ and compare this answer with the other answers.

This nearly equal problem demonstrates the influence of numbers that appear after the decimal point, but if you are curious about the influence of such numbers, set up problems that involve "nearly equal" examples, do the calculations with and without "rounding off" numbers, and compare the results.

This kind of mathematical exercise will help you become more comfortable with how the numbers in these problems work and will help you develop your confidence in doing mathematics of radiographic exposure calculations.

Problem 7: This problem is a REVERSAL problem.

TECHNIQUE 13	change to	TECHNIQUE 14
75 kVp		75 kVp
800 mA		_____ mA
0.025 sec		0.05 sec
20 mAs		_____ mAs
5:1 Focused Grid		8:1 Focused Grid
72″ SID		50″ SID
Screen Speed 250		Screen Speed 250

Your final solution to this technique should match part of Problem 6. You will need to do the problem to discover which part of Problem 6 gives the match.

PROCEDURE:

Again, do the following,

1. List the technique changes.

2. Write formulas and extract vital information.

3. Show calculations.

Technique changes include:

- mA

- mAs

- grid ratio change

- Distance change

Step 1: Write the formula for MA.

$$mA = \frac{mAs}{Time}$$

Step 2: Extract the vital information by using the information in Technique 13 as a starting point.

$$mA = X$$

$$Exposure\ Time = 0.05\ sec$$

$$mAs = 20$$

Step 3: Set up the equation and complete the calculations for mA. Do not use any shortcut methods.

$$mA = \frac{20}{0.05}$$

$$mA = 20\ divided\ by\ 0.05$$

ANSWER:

400 mA

Step 4: The mAs can now be calculated.

The formula is: $mAs = mA \times Time$

$$mAs = 400 \times 0.05\ second$$

ANSWER:

20 mAs

Your technique now looks like this:

75 kVp	8:1 Focused Grid
400 mA	50″ SID
0.05 seconds	Screen Speed 250
20 mAs	

Step 5: Next, compensate for a change in the grid ratio from 5:1 to 8:1. You will need to know the conversion factors for each of the two grids. It is assumed that both grids are adjusted for the nontypical SIDs used in both techniques. State the formula for the grid conversion and complete the calculations.

$$\frac{NEW\ Grid\ Factor}{ORIGINAL\ Grid\ Factor} = Conversion\ factor \times Original\ mAs$$

Step 7: List the Grid Conversion Factors and do calculations.

Original Grid = 5:1 Factor 2

NEW Grid = 8:1 Factor 4

$$\frac{\text{New Grid Factor}}{\text{Original Grid Factor}} \frac{4}{2} = 2 \times 20 \text{ (Working mAs)}$$

ANSWER:

NEW mAs = 40

The original mAs doubled because of the change to a focused grid with a higher ratio. Now we need to adjust either the mA or the exposure time to equal 40 mAs.

An increase in the exposure time may introduce motion unsharpness, so adjust the mA and leave the exposure time at 0.05 sec.

Do not adjust the kVp.

Step 8: Write formula for mAs and do calculations.

$$mA = \frac{mAs}{\text{Seconds}} \text{ (Exposure Time)}$$

$$mA = \frac{40}{0.05}$$

ANSWER:

800 mA

Your technique now looks like this:

75 kVp	8:1 focused grid
800 mA	50″ SID
0.05 sec	Screen Speed 250
40 mAs	

Step 9: The last technique change involves distance.

Step 10: Write the formula.

$$\frac{mAs_1}{MAS_2} = \frac{d_1^2}{D_2^2}$$

Step 11: Extract the vital information.

$$mAs_1 = 40$$

$$MAS_2 = X$$

$$d_1^2 = 72″$$

$$D_2^2 = 50″$$

Step 12: Set up equation and do calculations:

$$\frac{40}{X} = \frac{72^2}{50^2}$$

Step 13: Invert equation and liberate the "X".

$$\cancel{40} \cdot \frac{X}{\cancel{40}} = \frac{50^2}{72^2} \cdot 40$$

$$X = \frac{(50 \times 50)\,40}{(72 \times 72)} = \frac{100000}{5184}$$

ANSWER:

19.290123 or 19 mAs

Step 14: You will need to readjust your mA to equal 19.3 mAs or closest available factor, probably 20 mAs. Begin with the formula for mA.

$$mA = \frac{mAs}{Time}$$

$$mA = \frac{20}{0.05}$$

ANSWER:

400 mA

Step 15: Calculate the mAs:

$$mAs = mA \times Time$$

$$mAs = 400 \times 0.05 = 20 \text{ mAs}$$

ANSWER:

YOUR FINAL TECHNIQUE BECOMES:

75 kVp	8:1 Focused Grid
400 mA	50" SID
0.05 sec	Screen Speed 250
20 mAs	

Compare this technique problem to Problem 6, Techniques 11 and 12. Write a short report, minimum one page, and think about the following items:

A. The presence of any noticeable differences or similarities in the two problem sets.

B. The **REVERSAL** of this technique and the rules, theories, laws of physics, and so forth that make such a reversal of techniques possible.

CHECK THE CALCULATIONS:

$$mAs_1 : MAS_2 :: d_1^2 : D_2^2$$

$$40 \; : \; 20 \; :: 72^2 : 50^2$$

$$40 \times (50 \times 50) = 100000$$

$$20 \times (72 \times 72) = 103680$$

If you multiply **19.290123** $\times (72 \times 72)$, you will get **99999.997**, which rounded off equals **100000**.

RESEARCH PROJECT 4: THE FOCAL SPOT

From the following narrative, pick a topic or combine related topics if you want and write a minimum three- to four-page paper. Your paper should be written in your own words. Be sure to include bibliographic references.

In the last set of practice problems, the techniques were adjusted to compensate for various changes in grid ratio, distance, exposure time, mA, and so forth. One of the central themes of these problems was an efficient way to eliminate motion unsharpness by increasing the mA so the exposure time could be decreased.

1. Should you consider the effects of the size of the focal spot on the recorded detail of the image on the film when you are selecting or adjusting the technique factors?

2. What are the factors that determine the size of the focal spot?

3. How important are the **heat units** in the development of your technique?

4. What role does kVp × Exposure Time × mA play in the development of a technique? In answering this question, explain how heat impacts on the use of the x-ray tube.

5. Is the focal spot size more or less important than the speed of the intensifying screens? Explain and justify your answer.

6. How does the speed or type of film used in the procedure affect the geometric sharpness or unsharpness of the resulting image? Is it more or less important than the size of the focal spot or the speed/type of intensifying screens? Explain and justify your answer.

7. Describe and explain the construction of a stationary x-ray tube versus a rotating x-ray tube and how this difference in construction may affect the selection of techniques and focal spot.

RESEARCH PROJECT 5: RECORDED DETAIL

For nearly 25 years, experts have agreed that the recorded detail of the radiographic image is best maintained, at least in part, by using the smallest practical focal spot.

This remains a sound practice theory from a geometrical point of view, because some loss of recorded detail may occur as the actual focal spot size "blooms" or enlarges slightly when there is an increase in mA or tube current. (Burns, 1992; Carroll, 1993; Hiss, 1993; Selman, 1985; Thompson, 1979.)

In the folklore of modern radiologic technology practice, radiographers are often taught that on a radiograph, one cannot see any image on the film that is smaller than the effective focal spot size.

However, in a study conducted at the Mayo Clinic, researchers thoroughly evaluated this commonly held belief and determined that structures smaller than the focal spot can be imaged and seen on a properly exposed film. (Stears, Gray and Frank, 1989.)

Think about the following:

1. Would it be true that structures smaller than the focal spot can be seen on

   A. magnification study films?

   B. spot film exposures?

2. Would any of the following items have more or less effect on geometric unsharpness? Be prepared to explain your answers.

   A. Intensifying screens

   B. Size of focal spot

   C. kVp range: 50 to 75

   D. kVp range: 75 to 85

   E. kVp range: 85 and higher

   F. Milliamperage settings

   G. Timer Settings

Special Projects

General instructions for Special Project Papers.

1. Use your own words in the papers.

2. If you use exact wording from a source that exceeds one paragraph, be sure to use quotation marks and document the source. If you have doubts about the use of quotation marks for exact information taken from a source, provide the quotation marks *and* cite the source in your bibliography.

3. For convenience, use parenthetical citations, that is, (author, publication date). In the bibliography alphabetize by last name of the first author. Use standard bibliographic style. DO NOT number the citations in the bibliography.

4. You may use books or journals, and in some instances, information from the popular media may be acceptable (newspapers, magazines, and so forth.) If information from the popular media is used, it should not exceed two sources. This includes information gleaned from wire services, and broadcast sources.

5. If controversial information is important to the text of the paper, include it and state your opinion, based on what you have read. You decide if the controversy is valid or not, and include your opinion based on your research.

6. Find and use the most up-to-date sources of information for current information. If the information can only be obtained from historical or dated sources, such as the early history of a subject, use that citation.

Note: If you are using this workbook for self-instructional purposes, try to do these exercises as part of additional reading. You will find that both the exercises and the reading will be more interesting and easier to understand.

You are encouraged to develop a research paper about any of the topics in this book that interest you, and consider presenting the paper at one of your professional meetings and/or submitting it for publication. Your colleagues, patients, and you will benefit greatly from your efforts.

SPECIAL PROJECT 1: INDEPENDENT STUDIES IN TECHNIQUE CHANGE ADJUSTMENTS

1. Design four sets of technique changes using at least two changes in mA with corresponding time adjustments. Include the mAs information in the final techniques and describe why you think the technique will work. Provide documentation to support the rationale for selected technique changes.

2. Design four sets of technique changes and include multiple technique combinations. Two sets should involve changes in distance, grid ratios, and intensifying screen changes. Try not to duplicate the changes.

SPECIAL PROJECT 2: INTENSIFYING SCREEN STUDIES

Intensifying screens are an indispensable part of a radiographer's work. This project focuses on these accessory items.

1. Describe, compare, and contrast the various types of intensifying screens.

2. Identify and describe the kinds of materials used in making radiographic films and how these materials are selected or adjusted to accommodate for the various intensifying screen speeds.

3. Include information on how the exposure techniques used for screens and nonscreen holders differ and why these differences exist.

4. From the information you obtain, compare and contrast the levels of image formation with respect to geometric and recorded detail, including why recorded image definition may be better or worse with slower screen speeds or nonscreen techniques than with the faster speeds. Discuss, explain, and document findings and conclusions.

5. Briefly discuss the pros and cons of using intensifying screen techniques over nonscreen techniques.

SPECIAL PROJECT 3: RECORDING RADIOGRAPHIC IMAGES

Research and write a paper that describes the historical progress of recording a radiographic image on film from its early development to the digitally-recorded images. You might also include a brief description of radiographic film used for specialized radiographic imaging such as industry, dental, autoradiography, electron microscopy, mammography, cineradiography, and so forth.

Discuss the types and materials used, the pros and cons, and why the changes were either used or discarded, and if known, the companies involved in this work. You might discuss safety considerations of film, permanence of the image, preservation techniques, and recorded definition qualities.

This paper should also include information regarding processing methods and the changes that evolved as a result of the automatic processors. Other considerations in this regard are the significant differences between the types of film used for manual processing versus automatic processing.

Final Examination

Instructions: Calculators are permitted, but show your work.

1. At 36″ SID, the mR was 5. The mR was changed to 1.25. What is the new distance?

2. The distance was 40″ SID and the mR was 7. The mR was changed to 1.75. What distance must be used?

3. A distance of 40″ SID and 20 mAs was used for a specific technique. If the distance is changed to 72″ SID, what mAs is needed?

4. What is the square root of 1600?

5. If the mA is 500 at .05 seconds, what mA will you need to keep the mAs constant if you change the time to 0.5 seconds?

6. A time of 0.1 was used at 55″ SID. The distance was changed to 36″ SID. What new time can be used to keep the mAs constant?

7. For a technique, 10 mR at 48″ SID was used. The distance was changed to 72″ SID. What is the new mR?

8. What is the formula for the Inverse Square Law?

9. If Student A took six abdominal radiographs and Student B took nine abdominal radiographs, answer the following questions:

A. How many more radiographs did Student B take than student A?

B. Student B took _____ times more radiographs than Student A.

C. Student B took _____ (fraction) of the radiographs.

BONUS QUESTION: Student B took _____ percent of

the radiographs, while Student A took _____ percent.

10. When a number is written like this: 36^2, what does it mean?

11. 72^2 equals _____.

12. 200 mA was used at a distance of 36" SID. The time was kept constant, but the distance was changed to 72" SID. What mA is needed to maintain the original density on the film?

13. It was desirable to change from a 6:1 grid to a 12:1 grid. The conversion factor for 6:1 is 3 and the conversion factor for 12:1 is 5.

   What is the resulting exposure factor for this change in grid ratios?

14. The number in the top position in a ratio or a fraction is called the

   _____, and the bottom number is the _____.

15. For a specific technique, 20 mR was used at 40″ SID. The mR was changed to 5. What is the required distance for this change in mR?

16. What is the square root of the following numbers?

   A. 2401? _____

   B. 72? _____

   C. 1296? _____

   D. 5184? _____

17. Make the adjustments in the following techniques:

TECHNIQUE A	change to	TECHNIQUE B
80 kVp		_____ kVp
200 mA		400 _____ mA
.1 sec		0.1 _____ sec
20 mAs		_____ mAs
40″ SID		40″ _____ SID
Screen Speed 300		300 _____ Screen Speed
12:1 Focused Grid		12:1 _____ Focused Grid

What rules or theories make this technique conversion possible?

18. Make adjustments in the following technique for a) Screen Speed 150; and b) 36″ SID.

STARTING TECHNIQUE:

75 kVp   72″ SID

300 mA   Screen Speed 300

0.4 second   5:1 Focused Grid

120 mAs

ANSWERS:

<u>75</u> kVp   <u>36″</u> SID

_____ mA   <u>150</u> Screen Speed

<u>0.1</u> seconds   <u>5:1</u> Focused Grid

_____ mAs

19. Adjust this technique for a change from 5:1 focused grid to 16:1 focused grid.

STARTING TECHNIQUE

90 kVp   40″ SID

100 mA   Screen Speed 250

0.3 second   5:1 focused grid

30 mAs

ANSWERS:

<u>90</u> kVp   <u>40″</u> SID

_____ mA   <u>250</u> Screen Speed

_____ Sec   <u>16:1</u> Focused Grid

_____ mAs

How is the grid ratio determined, and why does this change impact on the need to adjust the technique?

20. Using the following problems, you are asked to evaluate and adjust Technique B, using Technique A as a starting point. Adjust mAs because of distance change; grid changes and increase kVp in technique B by 15%, and adjust all other technical factors in Technique B to accommodate the changes.

TECHNIQUE A	TECHNIQUE B
60 kVp	_____ kVp
500 mA	_____ mA
0.2 sec	0.2 sec
100 mAs	_____ mAs
72″ SID	36″ SID
6:1 focused grid	16:1 focused grid
100 Screen Speed	100 Screen Speed

Answer Key

Pre-test Answers:

1. A
2. C
3. Denominator
4. 2:24
   15:5
   24:12
5. A
6. C
7. A:B = C:D: x = 7.5
8. C
9. A DIRECT PROPORTION is a proportion in which one quantity maintains the same ratio to another quantity as the latter changes in the same direction.
10. An INVERSE Proportion is a proportion in which as one quantity varies, the other quantity changes, but in the OPPOSITE DIRECTION.
11. The INVERSE SQUARE LAW states: "The intensity of the x-ray beam varies inversely with the square of the distance."
12. A SQUARE ROOT is any number that when multiplied by itself equals that number.
13. The symbol for "Square Root" is: $\sqrt{}$
14. 55
15. A. 1296 B. 1600 C. 3025
    D. 5184 E. 10609

Answers for page 15: Distances Squared

1. $36 \times 36 = 1296$
2. $40 \times 40 = 1600$
3. $50 \times 50 = 2500$
4. $55 \times 55 = 3025$
5. $20 \times 20 = 400$
6. $72 \times 72 = 5184$
7. $28 \times 28 = 784$
8. $100 \times 100 = 10,000$
9. $(50 - 10)^2 = 40 \times 40 = 1600$
10. $(10 \times 10) - 50 = 50$

Answers for pages 17-18

1. E
2. A
3. B
4. A (TRUE)
5. C
6. D

Answers for pages 27-28

1. Ratios are fractions that indicate the relationship of one number to another. A ratio indicates how many times larger or smaller one number is to another number.

2. 5:10   OR $\frac{5}{10}$

3. The number that is being asked about.
4. How many times larger or smaller one number is to another number.
5. No.
6. Inches must be changed to centimeters, or the centimeters must be changed to inches. Ratios, as with most numbers, can be calculated only in the same units.

	With a colon	As a fraction	Lowest terms
7. 2″ is to 24″	2:24	2/24	1/12
8. Team A won 5 out of 20 games	5:20	5/20	1/4
9. 15 to 5	15:5	15/5	3/1
10. 24 to 12	24:12	24/12	2/1
11. If 5:1 Grid = 2 and 16:1 Grid = 6, change from 5:1 to 16:1 grid	6:2	6/2	3/1

	With a colon	As a fraction	Lowest terms
12. 1 ft to 36"	12:36	12/36	1/3
13. 10 min to 1 hr	10:60	10/60	1/6
14. 2 cm to 4 cm	2:4	2/4	1/2
15. 8 cc to 20 cc	8:20	8/20	2/5
16. 6 mR is to 20 mR	6:20	6/20	3/10

	Grid Ratio		Factor		Original mAs		New mAs
17.	$\dfrac{8:1}{5:1}$	=	$\dfrac{4}{2}$	=	2 × 30	=	60 mAs
18.	$\dfrac{16:1}{12:1}$	=	$\dfrac{6}{5}$	=	1.2 × 50	=	60 mAs
19.	$\dfrac{16:1}{8:1}$	=	$\dfrac{6}{4}$	=	1.5 × 10	=	15 mAs
20.	$\dfrac{6:1}{16:1}$	=	$\dfrac{3}{6}$	=	.05 × 2	=	10 mAs

Answers for page 37: Proportions Quiz

1. 8.4
2. 143.1
3. 12
4. 3.2
5. 3.75
6. 4.8

Answers for pages 42-43: Direct Proportion Problems

2. 38.58 or 39 mAs
3. .45 second or 9/20 second
4. 50 mAs

Answers for page 45: Direct Proportion Review

1. A **DIRECT PROPORTION** is a proportion, and as one quantity changes, the other changes in an equal amount; thus both proportions maintain the same ratio to each other. As one side increases, the other side also increases an equal amount, and as one side decreases, the other side decreases by an equal amount.
2. The other side **DOUBLES.**
3. A. mAs and Distance; B. mA and Distance; C. Time and Distance.
4. Subscript numbers are used to identify the numbers.
5. Superscript numbers (exponents) indicate how many times a number is to be multiplied by itself.
6. The number is SQUARED: $36 \times 36 = 1296$.
7. $A:B = C:D$ With a colon.

$$\frac{A}{B} = \frac{C}{D} \qquad \text{As a fraction.}$$

8. Small letters are used to identify **Original Factors.**
   Capital letters are used to identify **New Factors.**

Answers for page 51: Inverse Proportion Review

1. An **inverse proportion** is a proportion in which as quantity "A" varies, the other quantity, "B," varies in the **opposite** direction.
2. 1. Milliamps and Time
   2. Intensity and Distance
3. A. Decreases
   B. Increases
4. 0.1 second
5. 1000 mA

Answers for pages 55-56: Inverse Proportion Problems

1. .025 second (1/40 second)
2. 200 mA
3. 300 mA
4. Original mAs = 90; Exposure Time: 0.1; New mAs = 90
5. New mA = 100
   New Time = .05 (1/20) second
   mAs = 5

Your answers for page 59 are based on the results of doing the experiment.

The experiment is set up to help you better understand how the intensity of the x-ray beam is inversely proportional to the square of the distance.

It is important to understand this concept.

Answers for page 63: Inverse Square Law Quiz and Review

1. The **Inverse Square Law** states: "The intensity of the x-ray beam varies **inversely** with the square of the distance.
2. The formula for the Inverse Square Law:

$$\frac{i_1}{I_2} = \frac{D_2^2}{d_1^2}$$

3. The formula may be written another way, as long as the inverse relationship is maintained.

$$\frac{I_1}{i_2} = \frac{d_1^2}{D_2^2}$$

4. When the distance is decreased, the intensity of the x-ray beam is increased. Conversely, as the distance is increased, the intensity of the beam is decreased. Because of this inverse relationship, the technical factors must be adjusted whenever the distance is changed.
5. A = Halved
   B = Doubled
6. The square root of the distance.

Answers for pages 67-69: Inverse Square Proportion Problems

3. 120 mR/min
4. 2.5 mR/min
5. 10 mR/min
6. 30 mR/min

Answers for pages 69-71: Finding Distance with Inverse Square Problems

7. 20" SID
8. 72" SID
9. 36" SID
10. 28.28 or 28.3" SID

Answers for pages 77-82: Quiz

1. 72" SID
2. 80" SID
3. 64.8 or 65 mAs
4. 72
5. 50 mA
6. .04 (1/25) second
7. 4.44 mR/min

8. There are two ways this formula can be written:

$$\frac{i_1}{I_2} = \frac{D_2^2}{d_1^2}$$

OR

$$\frac{I_1}{i_2} = \frac{d_1^2}{D_2^2}$$

9. A. Student B took three more radiographs.
   B. 1.5 times more radiographs were taken by Student B than Student A.
   C. 3/5 of all the radiographs were taken by Student B.

10. "2" is the exponent, which means 36×36.
    The solution is 1296.

11. 5184

12. 800 mA

13. 1.6 (5/3)

14. Numerator
    Denominator

15. 80″ SID

16. A. 49
    B. 8.48

Answers for Final Examination

1. 72"
2. 80"
3. 64.5 or 65 mAs
4. 40"
5. 50 mA
6. 0.04 (1/25) sec (0.0428429)
7. 4.44 mR
8.

$$\frac{i_1}{I_2} = \frac{D_2^2}{d_1^2}$$

OR

$$\frac{I_1}{i_2} = \frac{d_1^2}{D_2^2}$$

9. A. 3
    B. 1.5
    C. 3/5

Bonus Question: 40%; 60%

10. 36×36 (The exponent means the number of times a number is to be multiplied by itself.)
11. 5184
12. 800 mA
13. 1.6
14. Numerator; Denominator
15. 80"
16. A. 49
    B. 8.5 (8.4852813)
    C. 36
    D. 72
17. 68 kVp; 40 mAs
    (A) The 15% Rule: Double the mAs; cut kVp by 15%.
18. 60 mAs. Adjust the mA or time to fit the new mAs. Suggest decrease in time to 0.1 second.

19. 90 mAs. Adjust your mA and time to fit the new mAs. Increase the mA three times and adjust the time accordingly if necessary. Do not change the kVp.

$$\text{A. } R = \frac{\text{Height of the lead strips}}{\text{Distance between the lead strips}}$$

20.
1. Change in distance. **Answer: 25 mAs**
2. Change from 6:1 to 16:1 grid. **Answer: 50 mAs**
3. Increase kVp in technique A by 15%. **Answer: 69 new kVp**
4. Adjust mAs by 1/2. **Answer: 25 mAs**
5. Adjust the mA to accommodate the new mAs. **Answer: 125 mAs**

YOUR FINAL TECHNIQUE SHOULD LOOK LIKE THIS:

69 kVp	36″ SID
125 mA	16:1 Focused Grid
0.2 second	100 Screen Speed
25 mAs	

Bibliography

Bressler EC: *Statutory credentialing of health care personnel*, ASRT Fellow Thesis, Albuquerque, New Mexico. American Society of Radiologic Technologists, 1981.

Burns EF: *Radiographic imaging: A guide for producing quality radiographs.* Philadelphia: WB Saunders Company, 1992.

Bushong SC: *Radiologic science for technologists.* Ed 5. St Louis: The CV Mosby Company, 1993.

Carlton RR, Adler AMcK: *Principles of radiographic imaging: An art and a science.* Albany, New York: Delmar Publishers, Inc, 1992.

Carroll QB: *Fuch's radiographic exposure, processing and quality control.* Ed 5. Springfield, Illinois: Charles C Thomas, 1993.

Cullinan AM, Cullinan JE. *Producing quality radiographs.* Ed 2. Philadelphia: JB Lippincott Company, 1994.

Hiss SS: *Understanding radiography.* Ed 3. Springfield, Illinois: Charles C Thomas, 1993.

Liebel-Flarsheim: *Characteristics and applications of x-ray grids.* Cincinnati: Liebel-Flarsheim Company, 1987.

Sperling AP, Stuart M: *Mathematics made simple.* Ed 5. New York: Doubleday, 1991.

Selman J: *The fundamentals of x-ray and radium physics.* Ed 7. Springfield, Illinois: Charles C Thomas, 1985.

Stears J, Gray J, Frank E: Radiologic exchange. ASRT *radiologic technology.* Vol 60. 429, 1989.

Thompson TT: *Cahoon's formulating x-ray techniques.* Ed 9. Durham, North Carolina: Duke University Press, 1979.

Recommended Resources

Barrows HS, Tamblyn RM: *Problem-based learning—an approach to medical education.* New York: Springer Publishing Company, Inc, 1980.

Bode A: Personal communication. Director of Radiologic Technology Program, Abbott-Northwestern Hospitals, Minneapolis, Minnesota, March 1992.

Bushong SC: *Radiologic science workbook and laboratory manual.* Ed 5. St Louis: The CV Mosby Company, 1993.

Dowd SB: Teaching strategies to foster critical thinking. ASRT *Radiologic technology.* 1991; 62:374.

Eastman Kodak. *The fundamentals of radiography.* Ed 12. Rochester, New York: Eastman Kodak Health Sciences Division, 1980.

Hiss SS: *A study guide to understanding radiography.* Ed 5. Springfield, Illinois: Charles C Thomas, 1993.

Jackson HL: Etter Lewis E, ed: *Mathematics of radiology and nuclear medicine.* St. Louis: Warren H. Green, Inc, 1971.

Meredith WJ, Massey JB: *Fundamental physics of radiology.* Ed 3. Chicago: Year Book Medical Publishers, Inc, 1977.

Stears John G, Gray Joel E, Frank ED: The three limits to prevent x-ray tube damage, ASRT *Radiologic technology* 1987; 58:423.

Trigg AM, Cordova FD: 1987. An integrated model of learning. ASRT *Radiologic Technology,* 58:431.

U.S. Department of Health and Human Services PHS/FDA. *The correlated lecture laboratory series in diagnostic radiological physics,* FDA 81-8150. Superintendent of Documents, 1981, Washington, D.C. Government Printing Office.

Developmental Testing Program in Radiologic Technology

Abbott-Northwestern Hospital. est. 1972. *Developmental Testing Program*. School of Radiologic Technology. Minneapolis, Mn. Abbott-Northwestern Hospital.

Information on this developmental testing program, developed and administered by Abbott-Northwestern Hospital in Minneapolis, Minnesota, is provided to let you know about another evaluation process.

This is a monthly 100-question test that measures objectives in radiologic technology. It was originally developed for the program at Abbott-Northwestern Hospital, and by 1992 some 200 radiologic technology programs and 1800 students across the United States were participants in this developmental testing program.

According to information about the tests, the questions include Technique, Anatomy, Positioning, Special Procedures, Radiation Protection, and Physics, and are changed or altered each month as well as on a yearly basis to keep testing materials up-to-date.

The questions are computer corrected, and results are mailed to participating program instructors. An excellent analysis of both the exam and the student's performance is provided with the corrected information.

This testing program is available through accredited programs in radiologic technology. There is a minimal fee per student, and the minimum subscription is for 9 months. The program is not available to graduate individuals or on an individual basis.

For additional information write to the Director of the Radiologic Technology Program at Abbott-Northwestern Hospitals; Developmental Testing Program. School of Radiologic Technology. Minneapolis, MN 55407. U.S.A.

NOTE: There are numerous books available that contain structured, simulated questions on various aspects of radiologic technology. Check with your instructor or your medical library, or check *Books in Print* for the names of current books.

Index